Practical Dermatologic Surgery

Practical Dermatologic Surgery

Edited by

RICHARD G. BENNETT, MD

Departments of Dermatology
University of California, Los Angeles
and
University of Southern California
Los Angeles, CA
USA

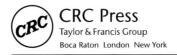

CRC Press
Taylor & Francis Group
Boca Raton London New York

CRC Press is an imprint of the
Taylor & Francis Group, an **informa** business

First edition published 2022
by CRC Press
2 Park Square, Milton Park, Abingdon, Oxon, OX14 4RN
and by CRC Press

6000 Broken Sound Parkway NW, Suite 300, Boca Raton, FL 33487-2742

© 2022 Taylor & Francis Group, LLC
CRC Press is an imprint of Taylor & Francis Group, LLC

Library of Congress Cataloging-in-Publication Data

Names: Bennett, Richard G., editor.
Title: Practical dermatologic surgery / edited by Richard G. Bennett.
Description: First edition. | Boca Raton : CRC Press, 2021. | Includes bibliographical references and index. | Summary: "Covering the full range of dermatologic surgery, this text will be essential reading for residents in dermatology, family practice, and surgical specialties needing to review a topic in detail. Each chapter is in brief, with tables, line drawings, and the essential references, offering an authoritative and up-to-date guide"-- Provided by publisher.
Identifiers: LCCN 2021011682 (print) | LCCN 2021011683 (ebook) |
ISBN 9780367511050 (paperback) | ISBN 9780367511098 (hardback) |
ISBN 9781003052432 (ebook)
Subjects: MESH: Dermatologic Surgical Procedures
Classification: LCC RD520 (print) | LCC RD520 (ebook) | NLM WR 670 |
DDC 617.4/77059--dc23
LC record available at https://lccn.loc.gov/2021011682
LC ebook record available at https://lccn.loc.gov/2021011683

ISBN: 978-0-367-51109-8 (hbk)
ISBN: 978-0-367-51105-0 (pbk)
ISBN: 978-1-003-05243-2 (ebk)

Typeset in Times LT Std
by KnowledgeWorks Global Ltd.

For beautiful Lisa

&

our wonderful daughters

Didi & Amelie

Contents

Section I   Dermatologic Surgery Background

Section II   Dermatologic Surgery Basics

Section III   Reconstructive Dermatologic Surgery

Section IV   Cosmetic Dermatologic Surgery

Preface

During the latter 20th century, a renaissance of dermatologic surgery occurred. Although dermatologists were initially at the forefront of skin surgical techniques in the early days of their specialty around 1900, a lag (1920–1975) ensued during which surgery became dormant in dermatology; at that time dermatology evolved into a medical rather than a surgical specialty. Fortunately in 1975, the first surgical journal in dermatology, the *Journal of Dermatologic Surgery*, appeared and has been published continuously ever since. There are now over 80 fellowships in Mohs Micrographic Surgery and Dermatologic Oncology overseen by the Accreditation Council for Graduate Medical Education (ACGME) and over 20 cosmetic dermatology fellowships overseen by the American Society for Dermatologic Surgery. Thus, almost one-quarter of dermatology residents take a 1-year surgical specialty fellowship after residency.

Many of the innovations in skin surgery that are now widely accepted were pioneered by dermatologists. For instance, hair transplantation, dermabrasion, and laser surgery were all first used by dermatologists. Perhaps the greatest contribution to skin surgery has been the development and expansion of Mohs micrographic surgery, which is a surgical/pathological technique for removing skin cancer. Many unique reconstructive techniques have been developed by dermatologic surgeons to close wounds after skin cancer removal. In addition, because dermatologists are required to have extensive pathology training during residency, they have been in a unique position to develop and advance this technique.

In the realm of cosmetic and aesthetic dermatology, dermatologists also have been at the forefront researching skin rejuvenation and expanding use of skin fillers, botox, and laser surgery. Because of extensive training in skin biology, dermatologists have a unique and expansive background to research cutaneous surgery.

The purpose of this book is to provide medical students and residents a practical summary of core knowledge in dermatologic surgery. The chapters are written by experts in each topic and presented in outline form that focuses on important facts and "pearls". Heavy emphasis is placed on historic development of dermatologic surgery as we feel it is important to understand where dermatologic surgery came from and where it is headed in the future.

Richard G. Bennett, MD
Los Angeles, CA

Acknowledgments

I wish to acknowledge the many individuals who contributed to this book. The American Society for Dermatologic Surgery (ASDS) helped to provide the impetus for this book through its Future Leaders Network. Both Catherine Duerdoth, executive director of the ASDS, and Tamika Walton, ASDS administrator, helped in the initial stages.

The bulk of the illustrations were done by Eo Trueblood, lead medical illustrator at Children's Hospital of Philadelphia. We borrowed some illustrations from a book written by myself in 1988 entitled *Fundamentals of Cutaneous Surgery*. These illustrations were done by Virginia Cantarella, now retired, but have stood the test of time. The front cover illustration was drawn by Dr. Mark Podwal, a dermatologist and artist extraordinaire. His drawings have appeared in the New York Times and The Metropolitan Museum of Art.

There have been numerous individuals who have vetted the chapters and to whom I am indebted. In particular, Jennifer Ledon, MD and Michael Xiong, MD, my previous fellows in Mohs micrographic surgery, Mark Juhl, previous resident in dermatology at the University of Illinois, and Dr. Jesicca Wu, a cosmetic dermatologist in Los Angeles. My fellowship coordinators, Danielle Urman and Kara Lukas, did most of the typing and research. Their unflappable attitude helped enormously to bring this book to the highest possible level of excellence. Lastly, I would like to thank Robert Peden of CRC Press for taking on this project. He kept me focused (not always an easy thing to do) and attended to numerous details I would never have imagined.

Contributors

Hina Ahmad, MD
Private practice, Walnut Creek, CA, USA

Brittany Ahuja, MD
Department of Anesthesiology, Robert Wood
Johnson Medical School, Rutgers University,
New Brunswick, NJ, USA

Murad Alam, MD
Department of Dermatology, Northwestern
University, Chicago, IL, USA

Mathew M. Avram, MD
Department of Dermatology, Massachusetts
General Hospital, Boston, MA, USA

Richard Bennett, MD
Department of Medicine (Dermatology), UCLA
School of Medicine, Los Angeles, CA,
USA
Department of Dermatology, USC School of
Medicine, Los Angeles, CA, USA

Jeanette M. Black, MD
Skincare and Laser Physicians of Beverly Hills,
Los Angeles, CA, USA

Alastair Carruthers, MD
Department of Dermatology and Skin Sciences,
University of British Columbia, Vancouver,
BC, Canada

Jean Carruthers, MD
Department of Ophthalmology and Ocular
Sciences, University of British Columbia,
Vancouver, BC, Canada

Steven Chow, MD, MS
Department of Dermatology, USC, Los Angeles,
CA, USA

Kyle Coleman, MD
Co-Owner, Etre, Cosmetic Dermatology and
Laser Center, New Orleans, LA, USA

William P. Coleman III, MD
Coleman Center for Cosmetic Dermatologic
Surgery, Metairie, LA, USA

Jonathan L. Cook, MD
Department of Dermatology, Duke University
Medical Center, Durham, NC, USA

Manish Gharia, MD
Medical College of Wisconsin, Milwaukee,
WI, USA

Mitchel P. Goldman, MD
Goldman, Butterwick, Fitzpatrick, Groff & Fabi,
San Diego, CA, USA

Allison Hanlon, MD, PhD
Vanderbilt University Medical Center, Nashville,
TN, USA

Derek H. Jones, MD
Skincare and Laser Physicians of Beverly Hills,
Los Angeles, CA, USA

Naomi Lawrence, MD
Department of Dermatologic and Cosmetic
Surgery, Cooper University Hospital, Marlton,
NJ, USA

Jennifer A. Ledon, MD
Bennett Surgery Center, Santa Monica,
CA, USA

Ken K. Lee, MD
Portland Dermatology Clinic, Portland, OR, USA

Austin Liu, MD
Department of Dermatologic and Cosmetic
Surgery, Cooper University Hospital, Marlton,
NJ, USA

Paul McAndrews, MD
Department of Dermatology, USC, Los Angeles,
CA, USA

Gary D. Monheit, MD
Total Skin and Beauty Dermatology Center, Birmingham, AL, USA

Tanya Nino, MD
Department of Dermatology, Loma Linda University School of Medicine, Loma Linda, CA, USA

Kapila V. Paghdal, MD, PharmD
Department of Dermatology, Northwestern University, Chicago, IL, USA

Silvina Pugliese, MD
Department of Dermatology, Loma Linda University School of Medicine, Loma Linda, CA, USA

Elisabeth K. Shim, MD
Private Practice Saint John's Medical Plaza, Santa Monica, CA, USA
Department of Dermatology, USC School of Medicine, Los Angeles, CA, USA

Teresa Soriano, MD
Division of Dermatology, UCLA, Los Angeles, CA, USA

Abel Torres, MD, JD
Department of Dermatology, University of Florida, Gainesville, FL, USA

Danielle Urman, BA
UCSD School of Medicine, San Diego, CA, USA

Ronald G. Wheeland, MD
Department of Dermatology, University of Missouri, Columbia, MO, USA

Michael Xiong, MD
Private practice, Myrtle Beach, SC, USA

Lisa Y. Xu, MD
Johns Hopkins Dermatology & Cosmetic Center, Lutherville-Timonium, MD, USA

Section I

Dermatologic Surgery Background

1

History of Dermatologic Surgery

Richard G. Bennett and Danielle Urman

Introduction

Dermatologic surgery is a subspecialty of dermatology that focuses on skin lesion removal, wound repair, and cosmetic procedures. Historically, dermatologists have made significant contributions to cutaneous surgery and have been leaders in areas such as Mohs micrographic surgery, laser surgery, tumescent liposuction, and soft tissue fillers. The following are what I consider the most significant contributions and contributors to cutaneous surgery. Additional historical information is found in many subsequent chapters.

I. Ancient History[1]

See Figure 1.1 for timelines.

A. Egypt

Edwin Smith Surgical Papyrus (c. 1800 B.C.E.) describes the use of cotton dressings, cotton sutures, and sandstone to smooth scars. Also mentioned is applying honey to wounds; recently, honey has been discovered to be antibacterial. Even today, honey is incorporated into modern wound dressings (MediHoney® Integra Life Sciences, Princeton, NJ).

B. India

Sushruta *Samhita* (c. 700 B.C.E.), an ancient Indian text, describes surgical instruments and skin flaps from the postauricular skin to the earlobe and from the cheek to the nose. Although the use of forehead skin as a flap to the nose (now known as the "forehead flap") is said to have been first done in ancient India, there is no documentation to support this legend.

C. Greece

Hippocrates (480–377 B.C.E.) discusses the use of heat cauterization and surgical instruments c. 400 B.C.E.

D. Rome

Celsus (25 B.C.E.–50 C.E.) describes the advancement skin flaps and ligation of arteries c. 50 C.E.

Galen (130 C.E.–200 C.E.) describes the placement of excisions, layered wound closure, and proper placement of incisions for advancement flaps c. 200 C.E.

Advances in skin closures were made by Galen working on injured gladiators in Pergamum in Asia Minor.

II. Renaissance

A. France

Paré (1510–1590) observes moist wound dressings to be superior to either dry dressings or allowing wounds to dry out, and in 1545 publishes this finding in "The Method of Treatment for Wounds Caused by Firearms" (Paris, V. Gaulterot).

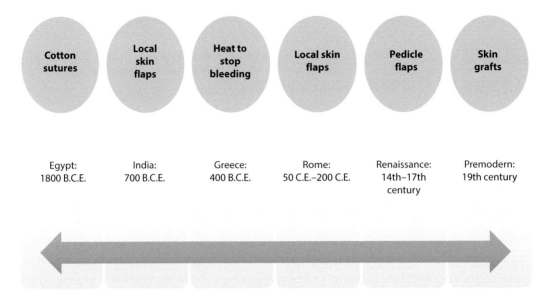

FIGURE 1.1   Timeline of major surgical developments from ancient times through the 19th century.

    B.   Italy

        Tagliacozzi (1546–1599) publishes in 1597 "De curtorum chirurgia per insitionem" (Venice, Gaspari Dindoni), which describes and illustrates open pedicle flaps to the ear and nose (Figure 1.2A).

III. 19th Century

    A.   England

        Carpue (1746–1848) publishes and illustrates in 1816 the open pedicle flap from the forehead to the nose (briefly reported being done previously in India in 1794) in "An account of two successful operations for restoring a lost nose from the integuments of the forehead" (London, Longman) (Figure 1.2B). This flap is now known as the "forehead flap".

> In the era before local or general anesthesia, the forehead flap described in 1816 by Carpue took 15 minutes to perform.

        Lister (1827–1912), a general surgeon, in 1867 describes using carbolic acid as an antiseptic on surgical incisions.

        J. R. Wolfe (1823–1904), an ophthalmologist, in 1875 describes defatting full-thickness grafts to enhance survival. To this day, full-thickness skin grafts are called "Wolfe grafts" in England.

    B.   France

        An intern, Reverdin (1842–1930), in 1869 describes the use of pinch grafts placed on wounds. Pinch grafts are small pieces (5–6 mm) of skin harvested with a needle and scalpel blade. The needle lifts up the skin and the scalpel cuts across it horizontally. These small skin pieces are placed on a granulating wound, which is then wrapped with a dressing for a week. Although rarely used today, this technique perhaps should be reconsidered.

        In 1872, Ollier de Lyon (1825–1900) describes the split-thickness skin grafts and the concept that immobilizing a skin graft leads to improved graft survival.

    C.   Germany

        Burow (1809–1874), an ophthalmologist, describes in 1838 the Burow wedge advancement flap for repair of a lateral lower eyelid defect. He also described Burow's solution (aluminum acetate dissolved in water), which is used today by dermatologists for wet to dry dressings on superficial wounds.

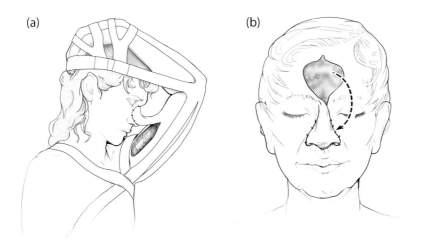

Italian method 1597   Indian method 1794

FIGURE 1.2A AND FIGURE 1.2B First described method to reconstruct the nose, by Gaspare Tagliacozzi in 1597. A skin flap is used from the inner arm to the nose. This nasal reconstruction method became known as the "Italian method" or the Tagliacozzi flap. The earliest known example of forehead skin used to reconstruct the nose. Originally reported by B.L. in a 1794 English magazine, describing a patient in India, this flap was subsequently illustrated and redescribed by J.C. Carpue in his own patient in 1816. This nasal reconstruction method became known as the "Indian method".

Koller (1857–1944), an ophthalmologist, in 1884 reports the first use of local anesthesia (cocaine), which was applied topically on the eyeball. The psychiatrist Sigmund Freud (1856–1939) had previously suggested to Koller that cocaine might be useful topically in this location.

Thiersch (1822–1895) describes in 1886 a very thin split-thickness skin graft. Technically, the split-thickness skin graft described by Thiersch is thinner than that described by Ollier in France in 1872. Nevertheless, split-thickness grafts became known as Ollier-Thiersch grafts.

D. United States

Warren (1778–1856) in 1840 describes advancement and rotation flaps.

Mütter (1811–1859) in 1843 describes transposition flaps at Jefferson Medical College in Philadelphia. Mütter innovated large transposition flaps from the shoulder to the anterior neck to repair large burn contracture scars. These contracture scars were common in women at that time due to kitchen fires.

Warren (1778–1856) in 1846 performs the first public demonstration of general anesthesia at the Massachusetts General Hospital.

Dunham (1862–1951) describes in 1893 the tunneled pedicle flap from the lateral forehead based on the anterior branch of the superficial temporal artery for nose and cheek reconstruction.

In 1899, Bloodgood (1867–1935) and Halsted (1852–1922) introduce the use of surgical gloves in the operating room at Johns Hopkins School of Medicine. Halsted also introduces the idea of gentle handling of tissue, complete hemostasis, and precise wound edge approximation.

Surgical gloves originated as a treatment for hand contact dermatitis in an operating room nurse rather than a method to prevent wound infection.

Piffard (1842–1910) in 1870 reports use of a modified gynecologic curette that became known as the Piffard dermal curette. Wigglesworth (1840–1896), first chairman of the dermatology department at the Massachusetts General Hospital, also popularizes the use of the dermal curette in 1876. The dermal curette is further modified with a slender handle by Fox (1846–1937) in 1902.[2]

Keyes (1843–1924) introduces the skin punch in 1887.

Punch excisions were originally used to remove facial gun powder tattoos in American Civil War veterans.

IV. 20th Century (Table 1.1)

A. Cryosurgery

Although the dermatologic use of cryogenic liquid air was described by A. Campbell White at the *fin de siècle* in 1899, and further popularized by Whitehouse (1864–1938) in 1907, especially for skin cancer, its widespread usage was limited by difficulty obtaining such cold liquid air. Various dermatologists subsequently used other freezing-type substances, such as liquid oxygen, carbon dioxide snow (dry ice, −78.5°C), and carbon dioxide slush (solid carbon dioxide mixed with acetone or alcohol). Finally, in 1950, Herman Allington (1906–1999), a dermatologist in San Francisco, described the use of liquid nitrogen (−195.6°C) on cotton swabs for treatment of various benign skin lesions. Subsequently, both Douglas Torre (1919–1996) in 1965 in New York and Setrag Zacarian (1921–1998) in 1967 in Springfield, MA developed hand-held spray devices for liquid nitrogen that could be used successfully to treat skin cancers; these devices could achieve a deeper freeze than possible with cotton-tipped applicators. During the 1960s and 1970s, Zacarian was instrumental in researching the biologic effects of liquid nitrogen on normal skin and tumors.

B. Chemical peels[3]

The phenol peel for acne scars was developed in 1903 by George MacKee (1878–1955), Chairman of Dermatology at New York Skin and Cancer Hospital. In 1961, Tom Baker (1925–), a plastic surgeon in Miami, popularized his "Baker formula" (phenol 88% 3 mL, croton oil 3 drops, Septisol soap 8 drops, and distilled water 2 mL). Application of this solution to the skin became known as chemabrasion, but was not popular in dermatology due to systemic absorption that occasionally resulted in cardiac arrhythmias. Eventually,

TABLE 1.1

Major Advances in Dermatologic Surgery

Procedure	Dermatologist[a]
Curettage	1870 – H. Piffard, 1876 – E. Wigglesworth
Punch Excision	1887 – E. Keyes
Cryosurgery	1899 – A. White, 1950 – H. Allington, 1965 – D. Torre, 1967 – S. Zacarian
Chemical Peels	1903 – G. MacKee, 1961 – T. Baker[e], 1962 – S. Ayres, 1980 – S. Stegman
Dermabrasion	1905 – E. Kromeyer, 1953 – A. Kurtin, 1955 – J. Burks, 1969 – N. Orentreich
Electrosurgery	1909 – G. MacKee, 1928 – W. Bovie[b]
Hair Transplantation	1929 – M. Sasakawa, 1939 – S. Okuda[d], 1959 – N. Orentreich
Mohs Micrographic Surgery	1941 – F. Mohs[c], 1970 – T. Tromovitch
Laser Surgery	1964 – L. Goldman, 1988 – R. Anderson and J. Parrish
Sclerotherapy	1985 – E. Bodian, 1987 – M. Goldman, 1988 – D. Duffy
Soft Tissue Fillers	1977 – N. Orentreich
Tumescent Liposuction	1985 – J. Klein
Local Skin Flaps	1989 – T. Tromovitch, S. Stegman, R. Glogau
Neurotoxin	1995 – J. Carruthers[d] and A. Carruthers

[a] Dermatologist unless otherwise indicated.
[b] Biophysicist.
[c] General surgeon.
[d] Ophthalmologist.
[e] Plastic surgeon.

in 1962, Sam Ayres Jr. (1893–1987), a Los Angeles dermatologist, popularized the use of trichloroacetic acid, a safer reagent than phenol. In 1982, Samuel Stegman (1939–1990), a San Francisco dermatologist, investigated the dermal effects of peeling agents and derm-abrasion on normal and sun-damaged skin. Although chemical peels are still used today, young dermatologists currently are likely to prefer using lasers to rejuvenate skin.

C. Dermabrasion[4]

   Dermabrasion was first used in 1905 by Ernest Kromayer (1862–1933), a German der-matologist who used motorized, rotating skin burrs. In 1953, Abner Kurtin (1912–1955), a New York dermatologist, resurrected dermabrasion using a rotary-driven wire brush along with ethyl chloride spray to anesthetize the skin.[5] Dermabrasion was further refined by James W. Burks (1911–1978) in 1955 and Norman Orentreich (1922–2019) in 1969, who developed a rotating diamond fraise or brush used after freezing the skin with refrigerants. Further modifications to help post-dermabrasion wound healing included preconditioning the skin before surgery with topical retinoic acid cream and the use of postoperative poly-ethylene oxide gel dressings (Stephen Mandy [1943–]). Although dermabrasion has been largely replaced by laser surgery, there are situations where dermabrasion is preferable.

D. Electrosurgery

   Dermatologists began using electrical devices for removing skin lesions in the early 20th century. MacKee reported in 1909 an electrical device to remove skin lesions, 20 years prior to when William T. Bovie (1882–1958) introduced his electrical apparatus into the operating room. Over the years, electro-surgical machines have evolved from the spark gap machines developed by Bovie to the solid-state machines used today. Currently, electro-surgical machines are generally used to stop bleeding, but other uses include scar modifica-tion and rhinophyma removal.

> Different types of electrosurgery were developed by W.T. Bovie, who sold his patent for $1.00 and died a poor man.

E. Hair transplantation[6]

   Hair transplantation was originally described by a Japanese dermatologist, Masao Sasakawa (1887–1932), in 1929. Two subsequent publications in the Japanese medical literature soon followed: one in 1939 by a Japanese ophthalmologist, Shoji Okuda (1886–1962), and another in 1943 by a Japanese urologist, Hajime Tamura (1897–1977). Unfortunately, World War II and the language barrier prevented dissemination of this technique. However, in 1959, Norman Orentreich independently developed the theory of donor dominance whereby non-balding scalp plug grafts (punch grafts) inserted into balding scalp plug holes retained the original donor graft characteristics, including growing hairs. Hair transplantation is now performed by the use of mini- and micrografts (much smaller than the original punch grafts) based on the concept of follicular units, giving a more normal-appearing hairline. It is interesting to note that the physicians performing hair transplantation today come from many different specialties besides dermatology, recreating what initially occurred in Japan in the first half of the 20th century.

F. Mohs micrographic surgery[7]

   Pioneered by a general surgeon, Dr. Frederic Mohs (1910–2002), at the University of Wisconsin in the 1930s, Mohs micrographic surgery (MMS) is the gold standard for removal of skin cancers. Mohs originally described using a tissue fixative (zinc chloride) paste *in vivo* and then removing and orientating the fixed tissue with subsequent compete microscopic examination of all cut surgical margins. After 1 week, the final layer of fixed tissue would slough off and the subsequent wound was allowed to heal by granulation. In 1970, the original MMS technique was modified by Ted Tromovitch (1932–1990), who eliminated the use of chemical fixative. Subsequently, in 1974 a successful case series with this modi-fication was published by Tromovitch and his colleague Sam Stegman; however, the micro-scopic examination technique remained the same. The new technique became known as the "fresh tissue technique", whereas the former technique with use of fixative became known as the "fixed tissue technique". Since the chemical fixative was no longer necessary, many wounds that before would have been left to heal by granulation and epidermization were now immediately repaired by skin grafts or skin flaps.

Mohs micrographic surgery is a surgical and pathologic technique that was described by a general surgeon (Frederic Mohs) but further developed by dermatologists because of their extensive training in skin pathology.

Today, dermatologists are the main specialists who perform Mohs micrographic surgery (now exclusively fresh tissue technique) because it involves both surgery and pathology. Surgeons, since they receive little or no training in skin pathology, cannot easily do this procedure.

G. Local skin flaps

Although mostly developed by head and neck surgeons, oculoplastic surgeons, and plastic surgeons, dermatologists became interested in local skin flaps with the advent of fresh tissue Mohs micrographic surgery. In 1989, Ted Tromovitch along with Sam Stegman and Richard Glogau in San Francisco published their local flap book entitled "Flaps and Grafts in Dermatologic Surgery" (Year Book Medical Publishers, Chicago). Since then, dermatologists have modified and developed new flap techniques to close wounds following Mohs micrographic surgery. For instance, in 1989, John Zitelli (1950–) helped to clarify the importance of angles with the bilobed flap.

H. Laser surgery

The use of lasers on skin was pioneered by Leon Goldman (1906–1997) in 1964 at the University of Cincinnati using carbon dioxide (CO_2) and argon lasers. Many subsequent lasers were developed by other dermatologists, e.g., the pulsed dye laser for vascular lesions in 1988 at the Wellman Center for Photomedicine at the Massachusetts General Hospital, under John Parish (1939–) and Rox Anderson (1950–), and more recently the fractionated CO_2 laser at the same institution.

I. Soft tissue fillers

In 1977, Orentreich reported an injection technique for microdroplet silicone. Injectable bovine collagen became available in the 1980s, but fell out of favor due to allergic reactions. Currently, there are many fillers available, consisting mostly of hyaluronic acid.

J. Liposuction

Liposuction was first described in the mid-1970s by Italian father and son gynecologic surgeons Arpad Fischer and Giorgio Fischer (1934–2001). The technique was originally done under general anesthesia, which was complicated by fluid shift problems and occasionally death when large volumes of fat were removed. A major breakthrough occurred in 1985 when Jeffrey Klein (1944–), a dermatologist, described tumescent liposuction; this local anesthetic technique allowed liposuction to be done more safely than when performed under general anesthesia. He described the use of a dilute local anesthetic infusion prior to liposuction, which enabled a large volume of fat to be removed safely.

Liposuction done with tumescent anesthesia avoids fluid shift problems that occur with general anesthesia. Fluid shift problems occasionally result in death.

K. Sclerotherapy and venous ablation

Sclerosing veins using polidocanol, saline, and other sclerosants was originally used in Europe, especially France and Germany, with American dermatologists Mitchel Goldman (1955–), David Duffy (1933–), and Eugene Bodian (1924–2010) at the forefront beginning in the 1980s. A technique called endovenous ablation, used by dermatologists in an outpatient setting for larger veins, uses catheters with either lasers or radiofrequency electrodes. The lasers target either hemoglobin (810 nm, 940 nm and 980 nm) or water (1320 nm and 1450 nm), resulting in heat damage to the vein wall collagen with subsequent fibrosis. Radiofrequency venous ablation uses controlled radiofrequency electrode on a venous catheter that causes collagen contraction and shrinkage of the vein wall diameter.

L. Neurotoxin

Botulinum toxin (Botox®) was developed in 1992 by a Canadian husband and wife team, Alastair Carruthers (1947–) (a dermatologist) and Jean Carruthers (1951–) (an oculoplastic surgeon), to reduce wrinkles in certain areas due to temporary paralysis of underlying muscles attached to the dermis. Jean Carruthers noticed that patients who received botulinum toxin injections for ocular diseases had reduced wrinkling in the glabella. Its extended use for sweat reduction in the palms and axilla was pioneered by dermatologists in Austria (1997) and in the United States (1998) (Richard Glogau [1947–], San Francisco).

Conclusion

Cutaneous surgery has evolved over many centuries. In modern times, dermatologists are at the forefront of cutaneous surgery, innovation, and expertise. It should be noted that other specialists have made significant contributions as well. Because there is growing interest in dermatologic surgery, further research and advances will be inevitable.

REFERENCES

1. Bennett RG. Fundamentals of Cutaneous Surgery. The C.V. Mosby Co, St. Louis, 1988; p. 3–16.
2. Bennett RG, Krull EA. ASDS 20th Anniversary: The History of Dermatologic Surgery. J Dermatol Surg Onc 1990; 16: 384–388.
3. Coleman W, Hanke W, Orentreich N et al. A History of Dermatologic Surgery in the United States. Dermatol Surg 2000; 26: 5–11.
4. Lawrence N, Mandy S, Yarborough J, Alt T. History of Dermabrasion. Dermatol Surg 2000; 26: 95–101.
5. Crissey JT, Parish LC, Holubar K. Historical Atlas of Dermatology and Dermatologists. The Parthenon Publishing Group, New York, 2002; p. 160.
6. Pak JP, Gazoni P, Zeballos A, Rassman W. The History of Hair Transplantation. Am J Cosmetic Surg 2008; 25: 231–236.
7. Brodland DG, Amonette R, Hanke W, Robins P. The History and Evolution of Mohs Micrographic Surgery. Dermatol Surg 2000; 26: 303–307.

2

Preoperative Evaluation and Avoiding Surgical Problems

Elisabeth K. Shim

Introduction

Dermatologic procedures can range from the minor and minimally invasive, such as a skin biopsy or laser surgery, to the more complicated and deeply invasive, such as a large excision, Mohs micrographic surgery, or tumescent liposuction. Because this specialty requires broad training in medical, surgical, and pathological aspects of skin disease, dermatologists are in a unique position to understand the risks and complications of cutaneous procedures.

Regardless of the complexity of a planned procedure, it is important to obtain a thorough history and description of the dermatologic problem pertinent to the procedure, to note current and past medical problems, to review the patient's list of medications and drug allergies, and to know the risks and complications of the procedure. Communicating with the patient to obtain a medical history and to discuss risks, complications, and alternative treatments is essential for avoiding complications. In addition, communication among staff is key to avoiding surgical errors.

The following illustrates the elements of an ideal history and physical examination obtained when evaluating a patient for the first time:

I. History of the Dermatologic Problem

  A. Problem duration.

  B. Associated symptoms: pain, pruritus, bleeding, tingling, or numbness (the last may be a symptom of perineural invasion by skin cancers).

  C. Previous treatment: recurrence/persistence after or failure of previous treatments.

  D. History of prior trauma.

  E. History of radiation: previously irradiated skin may be more apt to scar and slow to heal; with previously irradiated tumors, there may be skip areas and high recurrence rates.

  F. History of infection: active or chronically infected areas may be more apt to scar, cysts may be apt to recur, and herpes simplex virus lesions may be activated by surgery.

II. Past Medical History

  A. Hematologic problems

    1. Anticoagulants

      a. Cardiovascular history: patients with a history of atrial fibrillation, cardiac stents, cerebral vascular accident, transient ischemic attack, or deep venous thrombosis are likely to be on prescription anticoagulants or aspirin.

      b. Anticoagulants and antiplatelet therapy: patients taking these should not stop their medications prior to dermatologic surgery. There have been anecdotal reports of the newer anticoagulants such as apixiban (Eliquis®), when used in combination with antiplatelet therapy such as clopidogrel (Plavix®), causing prolonged bleeding intraoperatively and postoperatively. Guidelines for perioperatively managing these combinations of drugs in dermatologic surgery are not currently available.

    c. Non-prescription supplements: some of these have anticoagulant effects, e.g., St. John's Wort, garlic, gingko biloba, ginger, ginseng, and vitamin E.

2. Low platelets: for cutaneous procedures, a platelet count of 50,000 per microliter is the minimum generally accepted as safe.

3. Anemia.

4. Bleeding disorders, e.g., von Willebrand's disease or Factor V deficiency.

5. History of prolonged bleeding during or after prior surgeries.

6. Prior transfusions: patients who have a history of transfusions may be at risk for prolonged bleeding with dermatologic surgery procedures.

> Patients who have a history of bleeding problems during or after prior surgeries are at risk of having prolonged bleeding with dermatologic surgery procedures.

7. Leukemia: chronic lymphocytic leukemia has a high rate of recurrence for both basal cell carcinomas and squamous cell carcinomas, as well as a higher rate of metastasis.[1]

B. Artificial implants

1. Artificial knees and hips: preoperative antibiotic prophylaxis is required if implanted within the past 2 years. Prophylaxis should always be considered in patients also with immunosuppression or diabetes, and in the case of inflammatory skin disease; sites such as the lower leg, oral mucosa, and groin; and repairs of the ear and nose. No prophylaxis is needed for plates or screws.[2]

2. Heart valves: patients with an artificial or porcine heart valve require preoperative antibiotic prophylaxis for their lifetimes. One hour prior to the procedure, amoxicillin 2 g or cephalexin 2 g is usually given. Clindamycin 600 mg, azithromycin 500 mg, or clarithromycin 500 mg can be given for patients allergic to penicillin.

3. Breast implants: special care is needed to not puncture the implant during local anesthesia or surgery in the breast area.

4. Vascular stents: usually do not require preoperative antibiotics.

C. Cardiac problems

1. Pacemaker: at the time of surgery, only short bursts of high-frequency electrosurgical currents should be used. Interference is more likely when using monoterminal than biterminal high-frequency electrosurgery.[3] Avoid using high-frequency electrosurgery near the pacemaker.

2. Defibrillator: high-frequency electrosurgical currents cannot be used; consider electrocautery (transference of heat only) or pressure.[3] Another alternative would be to have a cardiologist or the manufacturer temporarily disable the defibrillator with a magnet and monitor the patient's heart rate and rhythm during surgery.

3. Arrhythmias or history of coronary artery disease: use a low concentration of epinephrine (1:200,000 or less), or no epinephrine. Patients over the age of 40 undergoing prolonged, invasive procedures that require large doses of local anesthetic, such as tumescent liposuction, should obtain clearance from their primary care provider or preferably their cardiologist, usually involving at minimum an electrocardiogram.

4. Heart murmur with regurgitation or history of rheumatic fever: preoperative antibiotic prophylaxis is required, especially with clinically infected wounds and mucosal procedures.

D. History of hypertension, cerebral vascular accident, or transient ischemic attacks: use of low epinephrine concentrations (1:200,000 or less) is advisable. Patients who are discovered to have undiagnosed malignant hypertension (systolic 180–200 mm Hg and diastolic 110–120 mm Hg) should have their procedures postponed until blood pressure is lowered by anti-hypertensive medications. Thus, it is important that all patients have their blood pressure taken during the initial visit.

E. Lung disease

   1. Current tobacco use: may influence vascular supply to flaps and grafts, especially if smoking more than two packs a day.[4] Although it may be unrealistic to expect a patient to completely cease tobacco use, it is important to discuss the increased risk of poor surgical outcomes associated with tobacco use and to encourage less use prior to surgery and during the healing period.

   2. Oxygen dependence: for patients who use supplemental oxygen, the flow is turned off during the use of electrosurgery. Patients who may not tolerate long procedures without oxygen, such as surgical reconstruction after Mohs micrographic surgery, usually know how long they can go without supplemental oxygen.

      a. Flammability: oxygen flow is prohibited in the presence of electrosurgical currents and lasers that may produce sparks.

      b. Pulse oximetry monitoring: may be advisable for prolonged procedures.

      c. Wound healing: may be prolonged due to poor tissue oxygenation.

F. History of tuberculosis: patients may have been exposed to an excessive number of x-rays or fluoroscopies, leading to skin cancers.

G. Liver disease

   1. Hepatic dysfunction: due to the decreased synthesis of vitamin K-dependent clotting factors (factors II [prothrombin], VII, IX, X, protein C, and protein S), hepatic dysfunction such as cirrhosis can be associated with prolonged bleeding. In these patients, it is best to avoid antibiotics that are metabolized by the liver.

      For a patient with history of hepatitis, especially hepatitis C, it is important to take precautions against accidental exposure to the patient's blood.

   2. Hepatitis, especially hepatitis C: precautions need to be taken to prevent exposure of healthcare personnel to body fluids, and special caution is necessary during instrument cleaning and sterilization. The physician or facility should have a protocol in place for Occupational Safety and Health Administration (OSHA) training of new personnel on concerns with blood-borne pathogens, including accidental exposures (e.g., needlestick injuries, blood splatters to the eyes, cuts from surgical blades and skin hooks). New patient care personnel should be up-to-date in their hepatitis B vaccinations. Useful methods of alerting personnel to hepatitis patients include adding biohazard stickers to Mohs maps and surgical trays, and flagging their electronic charts.

H. Kidney disease: patients with kidney disease may not normally excrete amide local anesthetics or antibiotics; therefore, it may be advisable to reduce dosages when using these.

I. Other infectious diseases

   1. Human immunodeficiency virus (HIV): patients who test positive for HIV may have great risk for infection and development of skin cancer with subsequent metastases. As with hepatitis C patients, it is essential to follow OSHA guidelines for the prevention of exposure to blood-borne pathogens, as well as to have a protocol in place for accidental exposure. Useful methods of alerting personnel to HIV positive patients include adding biohazard stickers to Mohs maps and surgical trays, and flagging their electronic charts.

   2. Herpes simplex virus (HSV): for patients with a history of recurrent HSV, it may be necessary to premedicate for chemical peels, laser procedures, surgeries around the mouth, or full-face procedures in order to avoid risk of viral activation with subsequent

auto-inoculation and possible scarring. Ideally, prophylaxis should begin 1 day prior to the procedure and consist of valacyclovir (Valtrex®) 500 mg by mouth twice daily for at least 3 days. Longer regimens (up to 14 days) have been recommended depending on the procedure and time to re-epithelialize.[5]

3. History of methicillin-resistant *Staphylococcus aureus* (MRSA): consider using a prophylactic topical and/or oral antibiotic with anti-MRSA efficacy. Some surgeons recommend application of mupirocin (Bactroban®), an ointment with anti-MRSA activity, to the nasal vestibules each night for 1–3 days prior to surgery. The patient can also undergo a nasopharyngeal swab and subsequent culture to check for MRSA presence prior to the procedure. Mupirocin ointment can be irritating if applied to open wounds, and its effects can be confused with infection and an allergic contact dermatitis. This can be avoided by diluting the mupirocin ointment with petrolatum ointment; however, a mupirocin/petrolatum mixture should not be used as a primary treatment for a known MRSA infection. Suspected infections should have a swab sent for culture and sensitivity testing. Judicious use of antibiotics, especially oral, is good medical practice to avoid creating antibiotic resistance.

> Patients with a history of MRSA infections are more likely to develop an MRSA infection postoperatively.

4. History of bacterial endocarditis, congenital heart defects, or surgically constructed pulmonary shunts/conduits: such patients may require antibiotic prophylaxis if the planned dermatologic procedure is in an area of infected skin or high-risk areas for infection, such as oral or nasal mucosa, groin, or below the knee.

J. Diabetes mellitus: poor glucose control interferes with wound healing and increases the risk of infection. There may also be a risk of hypoglycemia with prolonged procedures, which can result in the patient becoming unconscious.

K. Thyroid disease: if hyperthyroidism is present, the patient may be more sensitive to epinephrine.

L. Pregnancy: avoid non-essential skin procedures, especially during the first two trimesters. If a skin biopsy or surgery is necessary, e.g., for melanoma, the treating physician should get written clearance from the patient's obstetrician prior to any procedure, and the use of epinephrine should be avoided.

M. History of vasovagal syncope ("fainting"): the physician should be comfortable dealing with syncope because this is one of the most common complications that can happen in a dermatologist's office, even with a routine skin biopsy.[6] If allowed, the patient should eat a proper meal prior to any procedure. Avoid performing procedures in the upright position if possible, even skin biopsies. If fainting occurs, it is important to either lay the patient flat with the legs elevated or place the operating table in the Trendelenburg position. All medical personnel should be current in Basic Life Support (BLS) training, and physicians should consider Advanced Cardiac Life Support (ACLS) training, especially if there is no reliably quick access to emergency care.[7]

N. History of organ transplantation: due to use of multiple immunomodulating drugs, patients with transplanted organs may be at high risk for development of numerous and aggressive skin cancers and metastases. Cardiac transplant recipients are at high risk of developing endocarditis and should be given preoperative prophylactic antibiotics.[5]

O. Prior problems with local anesthesia

1. Stated "allergy" to epinephrine: these patients often had episodes of tachycardia or a feeling of impending doom from the use of high epinephrine doses or from inadvertent arterial injections during prior procedures. Nonetheless, these reactions should be taken seriously, and the use of epinephrine is not advisable. When injecting a local

anesthetic with epinephrine in a highly vascular area of the face, drawing back prior to injection is important to avoid an intra-arterial injection that may elicit an adverse reaction.

2. Stated allergy to local anesthesia: these patients usually are allergic to preservatives (especially para-amino benzoic acid) in the anesthetic solution. Such a patient might undergo an evaluation with an allergist prior to any procedure in which a local anesthetic is used. If the patient is only allergic to preservatives, preservative-free lidocaine (Xylocaine®), mepivacaine (Carbocaine®), and bupivacaine (Marcaine®) can be used. Compared to lidocaine, bupivacaine has a slower onset of action but longer duration; it also has a risk of causing heart arrhythmias.

3. Stated allergy to all local anesthetic agents: for these patients, injectable normal saline or diphenhydramine (Benadryl®) can be used as alternatives. However, the dosage limits of diphenhydramine may pose a problem, making it useful only for very small procedures such as skin biopsies or small excisions. Another alternative would be to try an amide anesthetic other than lidocaine, such as mepivacaine or bupivacaine, if allergy tests fail to confirm allergy to these agents.

P. History of hypertrophic scars or keloids

1. Hypertrophic scars: a history of hypertrophic scars has little meaning, as these scars usually result from wound healing where the wound is under extreme tension.

2. Keloids: a history of keloids puts the patient at great risk of developing a future keloid with any procedure. However, keloids in the central face are rare, if they occur at all.

3. Oral retinoids: if the patient recently used oral retinoids, e.g., isotretinoin (Accutane®), then excess scarring can occur. Avoid ablative or invasive procedures for 2 years after discontinuation of this medication.

Q. History of double-jointedness: in patients with this condition, scars tend to spread.

III. Medication Allergies and List of Current Medications

A. Documentation: essential to avoid complications such as anaphylaxis, rash, and medication interactions.

IV. Personal and Family Cancer History

A. Skin cancer: patients with a history of skin cancer, notably multiple family members with melanoma or dysplastic nevi, may have increased risk of melanoma development.

B. Other cancers: internal malignancies may be associated with many dermatologic problems, e.g., Muir-Torre syndrome and Cowden disease.

V. Social History

A. Occupation and work history: factors associated with the patient's work history, e.g., sun or chemical exposure, may increase the risk of skin cancer. If the surgical site or procedure is pertinent to the patient's function or appearance, he or she may need to know the expected "downtime".

B. Residential history and outdoor hobbies: where the patient was raised and any outdoor hobbies they have may be associated with an increased risk of skin cancer; e.g., sun intensity increases close to the equator and at high elevations. In rural settings, patients may be exposed to arsenic through their drinking water.

C. Home situation: understanding the patient's home situation may help with informed consent issues and with surgical aftercare, such as wound care.

VI. Physical Exam

A. General appearance

1. Well-appearing: very old, cachectic, frail patients with multiple medical problems and those who are wheelchair-bound may not be well enough to tolerate prolonged procedures, may have underlying undiagnosed medical conditions, or may have aftercare

issues (e.g., ability to perform wound care, transportation problems). These may affect the decision-making process when planning a procedure.

    2. Morbidly obese: due to their limited mobility, morbidly obese patients may have more difficulty with back problems, positioning for prolonged procedures, or wound care.

B. Vital signs

    1. Fever or signs/symptoms of infection: patients should not undergo a procedure if they have untreated active bacterial or viral infections, particularly in the treatment area.

    2. Blood pressure and pulse: if the patient is to undergo a procedure that is prolonged or requires a large quantity of local anesthetic, it is important to determine blood pressure and pulse preoperatively. Undiagnosed malignant hypertension (blood pressure >180–200 mm Hg systolic or >110–120 mm Hg diastolic) needs immediate attention and requires postponing the procedure until the patient's blood pressure is stabilized at a normal level.[8]

> Taking the patient's blood pressure preoperatively may reveal unknown malignant hypertension and save the patient's life.

    3. Weight: when a procedure requires large amounts of local anesthetic, it is important to note if the patient is thin and frail.

C. Lymphadenopathy: it is important to check the appropriate lymph nodes before treating aggressive skin cancers with a high risk of metastasis, including squamous cell carcinomas, melanomas, and pleomorphic sarcomas.

D. Pedal pulse: before operating on the feet, especially the sole, it is advisable to check and document the strength of the pedal pulse.

E. General skin exam

    1. Fitzpatrick skin type: pertinent to risks of skin cancer and complications from laser procedures, such as hypo- and hyper-pigmentation (Table 2.1).

    2. Modified Glogau classification: important to note before chemical peels or laser treatments (Table 2.2); indicates the amount of solar damage to skin.

    3. Previous scars, pigmentation irregularities, and large pore size (sebaceous skin): these features should be noted if in the surgical area, as their presence may affect cosmetic outcome and the risk of complications.

    4. Asymmetry: important to note prior to procedures involving the nose, mouth, brows, and eyelids, and for cosmetic procedures such as fillers or botulinum toxin injections.

F. Physical examination of lesion: in addition to location and size, dermatologists describe the lesion color, morphology, and surface texture.

> Description of a skin lesion should include: 1. location, 2. size, 3. color, 4. morphology, and 5. surface texture.

    1. Location: in skin cancer treatment, confirming the site is critical. Biopsy sites can disappear quickly, especially after a few weeks. It

TABLE 2.1

Fitzpatrick Skin Types

Skin Type	Color	Burning/Tanning Response
I	White	Always burns, never tans
II	White	Usually burns, sometimes tans
III	White	Sometimes burns, always tans
IV	Brown	Rarely burns, always tans
V	Dark brown	Rarely burns, tans easily
VI	Black	Never burns, always tans

TABLE 2.2

Modified Glogau Classification

Photoaging Type	Photoaging	Pigment	Keratoses	Wrinkles	Colloid Degeneration
I	Mild	No change	None	None	None
II	Moderate	Faint lentigines	None	Yes, with facial expressions	None
III	Advanced	Prominent lentigines	Visible	Yes, at rest	None
IV	Severe	Numerous lentigines	Visible and with malignancies	Yes, extensive	Mild
V	Very severe	Numerous lentigines and dyschromia	Numerous and with malignancies	Yes, extensive with secondary wrinkle lines	Extensive

is therefore important to take photos (at multiple angles if indicated) and/or to make precise diagrams with multiple landmarks. Using the patient's cell phone to take photographs of the biopsy location is compliant with the Health Insurance Portability and Accountability Act of 1996 (HIPAA).

2. Size: measure precisely and record in the operative/procedure notes.
3. Color: black, brown, flesh-colored, red, or telangiectatic (reddish with fine telangiectasias).
4. Lesion morphology
    i. Macule: small flat lesion, <1 cm (Figure 2.1A).
    ii. Patch: large flat lesion, 1 cm or larger (Figure 2.1B).
    iii. Plaque: large, slightly elevated, flat-topped lesion, >1 cm (Figure 2.1C). Often further described as indurated or sclerotic, meaning hard or firm when palpated.
    iv. Papule: small raised lesion, <1 cm (Figure 2.1D).
    v. Nodule: large raised lesion, 1–2 cm (Figure 2.1E).
    vi. Tumor: very large raised lesion, >2 cm (Figure 2.1F).
    vii. Vesicle: small lesion filled with clear fluid, <1 cm (Figure 2.1G).
    viii. Pustule: small, pus-filled lesion, <1 cm.
    ix. Abscess: large, red nodule, usually >1 cm.
    x. Bulla: large, fluid-filled lesion, >1 cm (Figure 2.1H).
    xi. Scar
        a. Flat.
        b. Atrophic.
        c. Hypertrophic: slightly raised, confined close to and within an incision line (Figure 2.2A).
        d. Keloid: raised, extends far beyond the boundary of an incision line (Figure 2.2B).
5. Surface texture or configuration
    i. Verrucous or verrucoid: wart-like, filiform.
    ii. Scaly: thin scales.
    iii. Keratotic: thick scales.
    iv. Smooth: lacks irregularities; may be pearly, pustular, or telangiectatic.
    v. Umbilicated: small lesion (<0.5 cm) with a dell in the center (Figure 2.3A).
    vi. Crateriform: large lesion (>0.5 cm) with keratotic center and elevated edges, either rolled or volcano-like (Figure 2.3B).

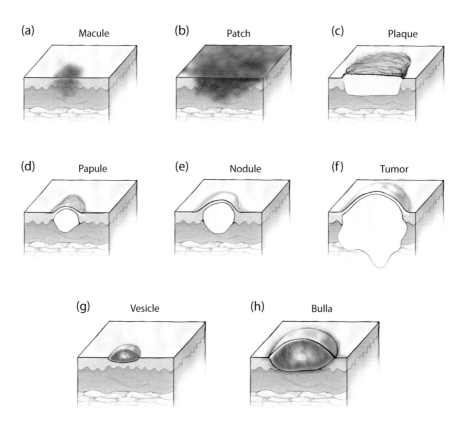

FIGURE 2.1 Primary skin lesion morphology. (A) Macule, a small flat lesion. (B) Patch, a large flat lesion. (C) Plaque, a large, raised, flat-topped lesion. (D) Papule, a small rounded lesion. (E) Nodule, a large rounded lesion. (F) Tumor, a very large and deep rounded lesion. (G) Vesicle, a small blister. (H) Bulla, a large blister.

      vii.   Atrophic: thin or depressed area of skin (Figure 2.3C).

     viii.   Excoriated: epidermis or surface of lesion lost due to scratching (Figure 2.3D).

      ix.   Eroded: superficial absence of tissue on top of tumor (Figure 2.3E).

       x.   Ulcerated: absence of tissue in a larger and deeper area (Figure 2.3F).

  6. Borders

       i.   Well-defined or poorly defined.

  7. Surface feel on palpation

       i.   Soft.

      ii.   Indurated: firm.

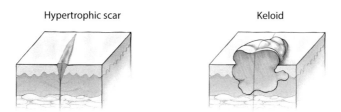

FIGURE 2.2 Comparison of hypertrophic and keloid scars. (A) Hypertrophic scar, a scar close to and within an incision line. (B) Keloid, a scar that extends far beyond the border of an incision line.

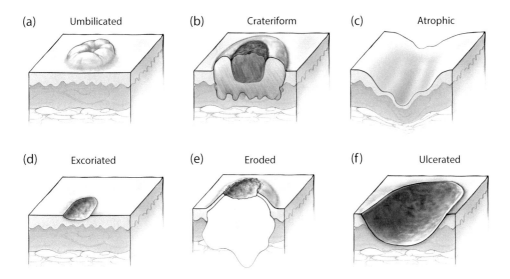

FIGURE 2.3 Surface lesion descriptors. (A) Umbilicated, a small central indentation. (B) Crateriform, a large tumor, often with rounded edges and central keratin core. (C) Atrophic, a depressed area of skin. (D) Excoriated, a small area of skin scraped away, often by fingernails. (E) Eroded, small area of epidermis and some dermis absent from the top of the lesion. (F) Ulcerated, full-thickness loss of epidermis and dermis over a large area.

        iii.   Ballotable: moveable when pressure applied to lesion between physician's index and middle fingers.

    8.   Location depth

        i.   Subcutaneous: has a deeper dermal component (e.g., subcutaneous cyst or lipoma).

VII. Medicolegal Considerations

    1.   Competency: is the patient competent to give informed written consent? Are there issues with dementia? Is there a power of attorney? Are there privacy-related issues in discussing the skin procedure and problem with a family member or caregiver?

    2.   Consent: signed informed written consent should be obtained for all procedures and photographs/videos. Prior to listing risks and complications, it is advisable to include the term "risks include but are not limited to". It is also advisable to have an attorney review the consent form. Some dermatologists do not routinely obtain consent for minor procedures such as skin biopsies; however, it is advisable that the treating physician use this at the discretion of his or her attorney.

    3.   Documentation: photographic confirmation of the skin biopsy site, and documentation with drawings and measurements can avoid wrong-site surgery, one of the most common causes of lawsuits in dermatology.

Conclusion

It is important to understand the descriptive terminology of dermatology and to take a complete lesion history. Details of the patient's present problem, medical and surgical history, and family and social history are essential to minimizing risks and complications, even with minor procedures. Expectations can be shaped and problems minimized by thorough communication with the patient as well as with ancillary staff.

REFERENCES

1. Weinberg AS, Ogle C, Shim E. Metastatic Cutaneous Squamous Cell Carcinoma: An Update. Dermatol Surg 2007; 33: 885–899.
2. DeFroda SF, Lamin E, Gil JA et al. Antibiotic Prophylaxis for Patients with a History of Total Joint Replacement. J Am Board Fam Med 2016; 29: 500–507.
3. Taheri A, Mansoori P, Sandoval L et al. Electrosurgery: Part II. Technology, Applications, and Safety of Electrosurgical Devices. J Am Acad Dermatol 2014; 70: 607.e1–607.e12.
4. Freiman A, Bird G, Metelitsa A et al. Cutaneous Effects of Smoking. J Cutan Med Surg 2004; 8: 415–423.
5. Wood L, Warner M, Billingsley E. Infectious Complications of Dermatologic Procedures. Dermatol Ther 2011; 24: 558–570.
6. Amici JM, Rogues AM, Lasheras A et al. A Prospective Study of the Incidence of Complications Associated with Dermatological Surgery. Br J Dermatol 2005; 153: 967–971.
7. Jiménez-Puya R et al. Complications in Dermatologic Surgery. Actas Dermosifiliogr 2009; 100: 661–668.
8. Bunick CG, Aasi SZ. Hemorrhagic Complications in Dermatologic Surgery. Dermatol Ther 2011; 24: 536–550.

3

Benign Skin Lesions

Hina Ahmad

Introduction

There are many benign skin lesions that a dermatologist evaluates on a daily basis. To diagnose these lesions, dermatologists are trained to correlate clinical morphology with histopathologic appearance and to categorize lesions based on their morphologic presentation and location.[1-3] With close clinical examination and occasional dermatoscopic examination, an experienced dermatologist can usually differentiate benign from malignant lesions. When the diagnosis is questionable, however, a shave or punch biopsy is warranted. The common benign lesions listed below are often treated surgically and categorized by surface morphology (see Figure 2.1).

I. Hyperkeratotic papule or plaque-rough elevated growths that arise from only the epidermis. These may be flesh colored, pink, brown, or black.

A black seborrheic keratosis may be confused with a melanoma.

   A. Seborrheic keratosis
   1. Tan to brown, rough, waxy "stuck-on" appearance.
   2. When black, may be confused with melanoma.
   3. Can occur anywhere on the skin except mucous membranes, palms, and soles.
   4. A sudden increase in number may be associated with internal malignancy (sign of Leser-Trélat).
   5. Usually requires no treatment unless the patient complains of pain, itching, or "irritation".
   6. Treatment: liquid nitrogen (Figures 3.1A and B), electrocautery, curettage (Figure 3.2), shave excision, 40% hydrogen peroxide gel (Eskata™).

   B. Verruca (wart)
   1. Smooth or filiform pink to tan papule and occasionally confluent plaque. May be multiple. In the genital and rectal regions, a wart is referred to as a condyloma and appears as a small whitish papule.
   2. Found anywhere on skin or mucosal surface.
   3. Caused by any one of several strains of human papillomavirus and therefore contagious, but poorly so.
   4. Treatment: liquid nitrogen (Figures 3.1A and B), curettage (Figure 3.2), trichloracetic acid, salicyclic acid, podophyllin, squaric acid, 15% sinecatechins ointment (Veregen™), imiquimod cream, 5-fluorouracil cream, intralesional interferon, electrocautery, high-frequency electrosurgery, photodynamic therapy, ablative CO_2 laser therapy, shave excision.

(a)   (b)

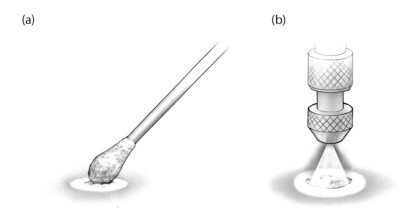

FIGURE 3.1A AND FIGURE 3.1B   Cotton tipped applicator applying liquid nitrogen to skin lesion. Note the halo around the lesion which is necessary for adequate treatment. Nozzle from spray gun used to apply liquid nitrogen to skin lesion. Note the halo produced around the lesion which is necessary for adequate treatment.

C. Epidermal nevus
   1. Tan to hyperpigmented linear or whorled plaques following lines of embryonic epidermal cell migration (Blaschko's lines).
   2. Congenital, therefore majority develop within first year of life.

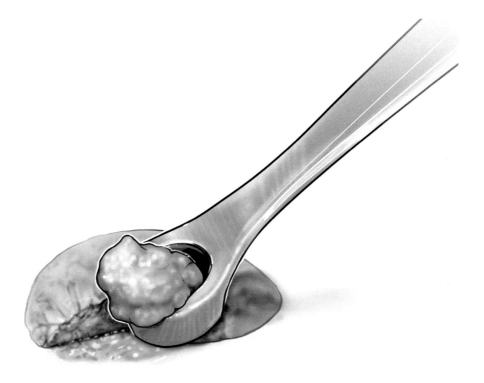

FIGURE 3.2   Dermal curette used to remove superficial skin lesion flush with the skin surface.

    3. Large lesions may be associated with neurologic or musculoskeletal abnormalities.

    4. Treatment: can be very difficult, but options include excision, ablative laser, or oral retinoids.

II. Smooth papule or plaque-fairly smooth elevated growth that has components arising from either the dermis alone, the epidermis alone, or both the dermis and epidermis (see Figure 2.1). The surface of these papules can sometimes have different textures. Color can vary and is dependent on what structures the lesion is derived from pathologically.

  A. Rosacea papule

    1. Pink papule typically seen on the central face and cheeks in middle-aged to elderly patients with underlying rosacea. Usually occurs with multiple lesions and then is referred to as acne rosacea.

> A rosacea papule can look like a basal cell carcinoma.

    2. If only one lesion, can sometimes be confused with basal cell carcinoma.

    3. Will resolve on its own over time or with treatment.

    4. Treatment: oral antibiotics such as doxycycline or minocycline, 15% azaleic acid topical gel, and topical antibiotic creams such as metronidazole cream or gel.

  B. Cherry angioma

    1. Bright red, dome-shaped papule typically seen in older patients on the arms and trunk.

    2. Fully or partially blanches with pressure.

    3. Consists of capillaries and post-capillary venules in the dermis.

    4. Treatment: electrocautery or high-frequency electrosurgery, laser ablation, punch excision, shave excision with electrocoagulation.

  C. Nevus (mole)

    1. Pink to brown, smooth, soft, dome-shaped papule, sometimes with a verrucoid surface. May have terminal hairs growing from it.

    2. Derived from epidermal and dermal melanocytes.

    3. If any change noted, especially irregular hyperpigmentation, a biopsy may be warranted to rule out atypia or conversion to melanoma.

    4. If hair growing from its center, the nevus may become "inflamed" because nevus cell growth surrounds and constricts the hair follicle.

    5. Treatment: shave removal (ineffective with some intradermal nevi) and excision.

  D. Congenital nevus

    1. Brown papule or plaque, often with mammilated or verrucous surface and terminal hairs. Seen typically at birth or within the first year of life.

    2. Classified as small (<1.5 cm diameter), medium (1.5–19.9 cm), or giant (>20 cm).

    3. Giant congenital nevi have a low (5–10%) but significant risk of developing melanoma. Melanoma arises deep within the lesion; therefore, any biopsy should be deep to detect malignant transformation.

    4. Risk of neurocutaneous melanosis with large midline or numerous congenital nevi.

    5. Treatment: observation. If change in pigmentation or nodularity arises, a deep incisional biopsy or an excision should be performed to detect deep malignant transformation. Serial photographs may be useful.

  E. Angiofibroma

    1. Also known as fibrous papule when it occurs on the nose ("fibrous papule of nose").

    2. Also seen in association with tuberous sclerosis where it occurs not only on the nose but also on the cheeks.

3. Flesh colored, smooth, dome-shaped papule. If solitary, may be confused with a basal cell carcinoma.

4. Pathology shows a localized area of fibrous and vascular proliferation in the upper dermis.

5. Treatment: shave excision.

F. Dermatofibroma

1. Tan, pink, or brown firm papule or nodule that feels fixed to underlying structures and is usually seen on the lower extremities.

2. When the lesion is pinched, a dimple is sometimes produced over the dermatofibroma, revealing a positive "dimple sign".

3. Etiology unclear, although thought to be often preceded by minor trauma like an insect bite.

4. May be pruritic.

5. Pathology reveals benign spindle-shaped fibroblasts in the mid to deep dermis. Rarely dermatofibromas can become large and invade subcutaneous tissue and even muscle.

6. Treatment is often discouraged.

7. Treatment: excision, triamcinolone acetonide (Kenalog- 10®) injection.

G. Syringoma

1. Small, usually multiple, firm skin-colored papules mostly around eyelids on both sides of the face. Rarely occurs on chest and vulva.

2. Clear cell variant can be associated with diabetes.

3. Adnexal neoplasm with ductal differentiation. On histology "tadpole" duct-like structures within the dermis.

4. Treatment: trichloracetic acid, liquid nitrogen, electrosurgery, laser ablation, punch excision.

H. Trichoepithelioma

1. Skin-colored papule presenting singularly or in clusters, typically on the face or chest, with a predilection for the nose.

2. Can be confused clinically and sometimes histologically with a basal cell carcinoma.

3. On pathology, follicular germinative differentiation is seen.

A trichoepithelioma can be confused clinically and pathologically with a basal cell carcinoma.

4. Treatment: electrosurgery, laser ablation, punch excision for solitary lesions.

I. Neurofibroma

1. Skin-colored, soft, and rubbery papule, often polypoid or pedunculated.

2. With palpation, can appreciate the "button-hole" sign, where an underlying dermal defect is appreciated in the area of the neurofibroma and the lesion can be easily invaginated.

3. If multiple, may be associated with neurofibromatosis.

4. Pathology reveals spindle cells (nerve cells) in a haphazard array within the dermis.

5. Treatment: excision.

J. Acrochordon (skin tag)

1. Small (1–2 mm), soft pedunculated papule either skin-colored, tan, or brown. Usually multiple.

2. Found most often in body folds like the neck, axilla, or groin.

3. When on neck sometimes catches on necklaces.

(a) (b)

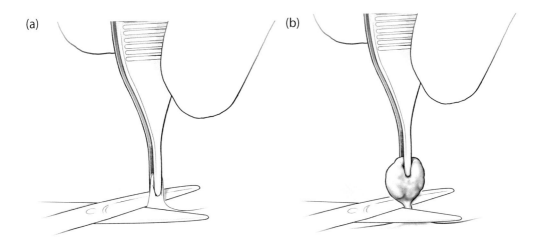

FIGURE 3.3 Using scissors to remove A. Skin tag (acrochordon) B. Fibroepitheliomatous polyp.

    4. Easily irritated and may become red, painful, and occasionally black (infarcted).

    5. Treatment: excision with scissors (Figure 3.3A).

K. Fibroepitheliomatous polyp

    1. Large, flesh colored, soft pedunculated papule with small stalk.

    2. Often occurs around the waist or inner thighs.

    3. Usually irritates patient by its presence.

    4. May become red and painful and occasionally black (infarcted).

    5. Treatment: excision with scissors (Figure 3.3B).

L. Sebaceous gland hyperplasia

    1. Yellow smooth papule, often with central dell, sometimes with overlying telangiectasias, seen most often in older adults on the central face.

> Multiple sebaceous gland hyperplasia on face may be associated with bowel malignancy (Muir-Torre syndrome).

    2. Can be confused clinically with basal cell carcinoma.

    3. Results from enlarged sebaceous glands within the dermis.

    4. If multiple, especially if seen with sebaceous adenomas, may be associated with large bowel malignancy (Muir-Torre syndrome).

    5. Treatment: electrosurgery, cryotherapy, laser ablation, shave excision.

M. Xanthelasma

    1. Smooth, round to oval, yellow to orange papules or plaques, usually on eyelids.

    2. If patient is young and presents with xanthelasma, a workup for hyperlipidemia is warranted although it occurs in less than half of the cases.

    3. Characteristic finding on pathology is the foam cell, which is a macrophage filled with lipid droplets.

    4. Treatment: trichloracetic acid, cryotherapy, laser ablation, excision.

N. Milium (plural milia)

    1. Small (1–2 mm), white, firm papule typically present on the face and seen in all age groups.

2. An early basal cell carcinoma can appear like a milium.

3. Use of moisturizers on face at night might promote development.

Multiple milia on the face are frequently associated with use of facial moisturizers at night.

4. Pathology reveals a small cyst with stratified squamous epithelial lining filled with keratin.

5. Treatment: incision of epidermal surface and extraction of cyst components, topical retinoids (if multiple lesions).

O. Molluscum contagiosum

1. Small (2–3 mm) umbilicated papules that are round and smooth.

2. Caused by DNA poxvirus.

3. Can occur anywhere on the skin but usually on face and genital area.

4. More common in children, especially on the face.

5. Considered a sexually transmitted disease when it occurs in genital area.

6. May become secondarily infected and if so have surrounding erythema.

7. Treatment: liquid nitrogen, curettage, remove top with syringe needle and express contents, cantharidin topically applied by physician.

III. Flat macule or patch-lesion derived from epidermis alone or dermal components alone.

A. Junctional nevus

1. Tan to brown macule with regular and well-defined borders. Typically symmetric with uniform coloration.

2. Any changes or irregularities in border, color, symmetry, or size should prompt a biopsy to rule out atypia or melanoma.

3. Pathology shows melanocytic nests at the junction of epidermis and dermis.

4. Treatment: excision.

B. Café au lait macule

1. Tan to light brown macule or patch, sometimes with irregular borders, usually on the trunk.

2. Typically congenital and seen in the first year of life.

3. If there are multiple, or large patches, may be associated with neurofibromatosis.

4. Pathology reveals normal epidermis with increased melanin content in the basilar keratinocytes.

5. Treatment: not recommended. Variable results with laser treatment.

C. Solar lentigo

1. Tan to brown, well circumscribed, fairly uniform macule, typically present on sun-exposed skin in elderly patients.

2. Small: usually 3–8 mm.

3. Progression to lentigo maligna melanoma has been debated, but any lesion that has irregular border, has enlarged, or has darkened in some areas warrants a biopsy.

4. Pathology reveals elongated clubbed-shaped rete ridges of the epidermis with an increase in basal layer pigmentation.

5. Treatment: cryotherapy, laser therapy, chemical peel.

D. Port-wine stain (nevus flammeus)

1. Red to violaceous patch that typically presents at birth and may fade in 1–3 years. May also become darker and hypertrophic with time.

2. Common location is the nape of the neck where it is commonly referred to as a "stork bite".

     3. Pathology reveals capillary dilation in the dermis.

     4. Treatment: pulse dye laser.

IV. Subcutaneous nodule – a growth in the deep dermis or subcutaneous fat which can be better felt than seen. There can be a variation in color with these lesions, but oftentimes the borders are indistinct and blurred due to the deep nature of the pathology.

  A. Lipoma

     1. Skin-colored, rubbery, mobile, deep, soft nodule that can be present at any site, with no overlying skin changes.

     2. If lesion is painful, it is more likely to be an angiolipoma.

     3. Pathology reveals a uniform population of fat cells in the deep dermis or subcutaneous tissue. However, the gross appearance of a lipoma shows large pale nodules of fat tissue.

     4. Treatment: small incision in overlying skin followed by pressure applied around lesion to push out lipoma. May first need to free up deep fibrous septal connections with blunt scissors.

  B. Blue nevus

     1. Dark blue to black indistinct macule or nodule.

     2. Can be present on any skin or mucosal site.

     3. Does not blanch with pressure. Can be mistaken for melanoma.

     4. Pathology reveals melanocytic nests deep in the dermis.

     5. Treatment: excision.

  C. Epidermal cyst (epidermal inclusion cyst, keratinous cyst, or infundibular cyst)

     1. Skin-colored to white, soft to firm, mobile nodule, usually with a central punctum.

     2. Most often seen on the face, scalp, and central trunk.

     3. Pathologically, an epidermal inclusion cyst has a capsule and is filled with malodorous, cheesy keratin. Although this type of cyst is sometimes referred to as a "sebaceous cyst", this term is a misnomer. A true sebaceous cyst refers to a steatocystoma cyst.

     4. Not to be confused with a pilar cyst (trichilemmal cyst) which almost always occurs on the scalp, has a very thick capsule, and has odorless, non-cheesy contents.

     5. May become red, swollen, and painful which indicates infection. When infected, avoid excision and treat with antibiotics. To provide immediate pain relief, one could consider intralesional triamcinolone acetonide (Kenalog- 10®) or incision and drainage.

     6. Treatment: excision when not infected.

  D. Hidradenitis suppurativa

     1. Multiple nodules (that are infected follicular derived cysts) in areas where apocrine glands are located especially in axillary, inguinal, and genital region.

> Any recurrently infected cyst in the axilla or groin is probably associated with hidradenitis suppurativa.

     2. Often recurrent and drain yellow to purulent fluid.

     3. If persist for months to years the cysts may extend subcutaneously and form epidermal-lined tracts or tunnels in the subcutaneous tissue.

     4. Around anus may progress after many years (about 30 years) to squamous cell carcinoma.

     5. Treatment typically consists of two antibiotics taken simultaneously (usually cephalexin [Keflex®] and trimethoprim/sulfamethoxazole [Bactrim], Keflex® and doxycycline, or rifampin and clindamycin [Cleocin®]) until draining ceases followed by complete surgical excision including all cysts, tracts, and scar tissue. For extensive disease adalimumab (Humira®) or infliximab (Remicade®) might be useful.

E. Keloid
1. Firm nodules, usually skin colored or slightly darker than skin.
2. Never seen in central face but often on earlobes, trunk, and upper arms.
3. Distinguished from a hypertrophic scar because it extends far beyond the lateral borders of the scar (see Figure 2.2A and B).
4. Pathology shows broad bands of horizontal thick collagen.
5. May recur with simple excision unless tension taken off wound edges at closure.
6. Treatment includes triamcinolone acetonide (Kenalog-10®) injections, excision using overlying skin as a flap to take tension off the closure. After keloid excision on the earlobe, pressure earrings may be helpful to prevent reoccurrence.

Conclusion

Given the large number of benign skin lesions, it is essential for physicians to be able to recognize key morphologic features that help categorize lesions. Through this methodology, dermatologists can usually differentiate benign from malignant lesions, although considerable overlap does exist. For this reason, it is essential to educate patients to see their dermatologist for any new or changing lesions, or for any lesions where the diagnosis is questionable. Most benign lesions do not require treatment unless they change, become symptomatic, or are disfiguring.

REFERENCES

1. Bolognia JL, Jorizzo JL, Shaffer JV. Dermatology, 3rd Edition. Elsevier Saunders, Philadelphia, PA, 2012.
2. James WD, Berger TG, Elston DM. Andrews' Diseases of the Skin: Clinical Dermatology, 10th Edition. Saunders, Canada, 2006.
3. Lebwohl MG, Heymann WR, Berth-Jones J, Couson I. Treatment of Skin Disease: Comprehensive Therapeutic Strategies, 3rd Edition. Saunders Elsevier, Philadelphia, PA, 2009.

4

Pre-malignant and Malignant Skin Lesions

Steven Chow

Introduction

Skin cancers are the most common malignancies. Although most individuals with skin cancers will not die from their disease, metastases and subsequent death can occur in a small number of patients. The three most common skin cancer types are basal cell carcinoma (BCC), squamous cell carcinoma (SCC), and melanoma. Ultraviolet radiation, especially sunlight, has been linked to skin cancer development, and its early detection allows for better survival and decreased morbidity.

I. Premalignant Lesions
   A. Actinic keratosis (AK)
      1. Rough (sandpaper-like) lesion, flat or slightly raised lesion. Can be flesh colored, pink, or sometimes pigmented. Often is more easily felt than seen.
         a. In highly sun-exposed anatomic locations (face, arms, and upper chest).
         b. Considered premalignant as a small percentage of lesions may progress to invasive squamous cell carcinoma. Histopathologically, atypical keratinocytes are present only in the epidermis.
         c. Patients with AKs have a propensity for developing skin cancers, as AKs are an indication of chronic and cumulative sun damage.
      2. Treatment: cryotherapy (liquid nitrogen [LN_2]) (see Figure 3.1), curettage (Figure 3.2), topical 5-fluoruracil (5-FU) cream or solution, topical imiquimod cream, photodynamic therapy (PDT), chemical peel, carbon dioxide laser.
   B. Cutaneous horn
      1. Horn-like projection above skin surface.
         a. Horn is comprised of compacted keratin.
         b. 20–30% of the time, a cutaneous horn overlies a squamous cell carcinoma (SCC), Bowen disease carcinoma, or a basal cell carcinoma (BCC).[1] Therefore, histological evaluation of the cutaneous horn base is important.
         c. 70–80% of the time, a cutaneous horn overlies an actinic keratosis or seborrheic keratosis.
      2. Treatment: excision or Mohs micrographic surgery if invasive malignancy (SCC, BCC, or Bowen disease carcinoma) is present at the base. If benign lesion at base, curettage or liquid nitrogen.
   C. Dysplastic nevus
      1. "Funny-looking" mole: an atypically appearing mole, usually with asymmetry of pigmentation, larger (>6 mm) than a normal nevus, with a poorly defined border.

2. Also known as atypical nevus, architecturally disordered nevus, nevus with melano-cytic dysplasia, or Clark nevus.

3. Often found in patients with multiple moles (>50). However, may occur sporadically in patients with only a few moles.

4. May be found in patients with a personal and strong family history of melanoma and multiple moles. This clinical combination of findings is known as "dysplastic nevus syndrome".

5. Biopsy may show scattered slightly atypical melanocytes and architectural disorder (bridging between epidermal papilla). Often graded as "mild", "moderate", "severe". Evolution to melanoma can occur and has been photodocumented. Thus, this lesion can be premalignant.

6. Patients with multiple moles and a personal or family history of melanoma should have total body photography so that any growth or pigmentary changes in moles can be documented.

II. Malignant Lesions

  A. Squamous cell carcinoma variants

    1. Keratoacanthoma (KA).

      a. A crateriform nodule or tumor with its central crater filled with keratin (see Figure 2.3B).

        i. Low-grade malignancy that can regress, but if it continues to enlarge, may invade underlying nerves, blood vessels, and may even metastasize. On central face may become particularly aggressive.

> Keratoacanthomas may invade underlying nerves and rarely blood vessels.

        ii. May be induced by sun exposure, a chronic scarring process, surgical trauma, a burn, or tar.

        iii. Currently considered a well-differentiated squamous cell carcinoma and should be managed as such.

      b. Grows rapidly: within 1–2 months. May regress spontaneously, especially if small.

      c. Treatment: excision, Mohs micrographic surgery, radiation, intralesional injection of either 5-FU, bleomycin, or methotrexate.

    2. Squamous cell carcinoma in-situ (SCCIS) non-Bowen disease type

      a. Small (<1 cm) scaly patch usually in sun-exposed areas.

      b. Proliferation of large keratin-producing cells that invade the epidermis only.

      c. Treatment: imiquimod cream, topical 5-FU, Mohs micrographic surgery, excision, curettage, CO_2 laser (if on lip), radiation, PDT.

    3. Squamous cell carcinoma in-situ (SCCIS) Bowen disease type (also known as Bowen disease carcinoma [BDC]).

      a. Erythematous scaly patch often greater than 1 cm.

        i. Usually on sun-exposed anatomic locations. If BDC occurs in non-sun-exposed areas, it may be associated with internal malignancy.

        ii. May be associated with arsenic exposure.

        iii. Large bizarre (bowenoid cells) and small atypical cells usually without keratin confined to the epidermis and external hair root sheaths.

        iv. When BDC occurs in the genital or periungual areas, it can be associated with oncogenic human papilloma virus (HPV) subtypes 16, 18, 31, and 35.[1] On the glans penis, Bowen disease carcinoma is known as erythroplasia of Queyrat.

      b.   Treatment: topical imiquimod cream, topical 5-FU cream or solution, Mohs micrographic surgery, excision, curettage, radiation, PDT.

B. Squamous cell carcinoma

    1. Second most common skin cancer type (basal cell carcinoma is the most common skin cancer).

    2. Erythematous scaly macule, patch, papule, or nodule. May be eroded or ulcerated.

    3. Often associated with excess sun exposure. Also associated with ultraviolet A (UVA) phototherapy treatment for psoriasis.

    4. Results from dermal invasion of SCCIS either BDC type or non-BDC type. If SCC evolves from non-BDC type, cells are large and keratotic; if SCC evolves from BDC type, cells are small and large atypical cells without prominent keratin.

    5. When Bowen disease carcinoma invades the dermis, it should be designated invasive Bowen disease carcinoma rather than invasive squamous cell carcinoma since its etiology and prognosis may be different.[2]

    6. Rate of SCC metastasis on all skin sites is small ranging from 0.5 to 5.2%.[1]

          a.   SCCs likely to metastasize have one or more of the following characteristics: >2 cm diameter, pathologic depth >4 mm, perineural invasion, vascular invasion, prior unsuccessful treatment, aggressive pathologic features.[3]

> Invasive Bowen disease carcinoma is a distinct type of squamous cell carcinoma to be distinguished from invasive non-Bowen disease squamous cell carcinoma.

          b.   Patient characteristics associated with SCC metastasis include immunosuppressed patients, especially those with chronic lymphocytic leukemia (CLL) and organ transplants on immunosuppressive medications.

          c.   High metastatic rates occur for SCCs located in scars or on the lip, ears, and scalp.

          d.   It is important to check for lymph node enlargement in the drainage area of all squamous cell carcinomas prior to treatment and at each follow-up visit.

    7. Treatment: curettage and electrocoagulation (C&E), or excision for small (<1 cm) lesions on the trunk and extremities. For large (>1 cm) lesions, excision, Mohs micrographic surgery, and radiation. For multiple small lesions, oral retinoids (Soriatane®), and capecitabine (Xeloda®) can be considered.

C. Basal cell carcinoma

    1. Most common skin cancer type in Caucasians.

    2. Associated with activation of the Smoothened (SMO) genes.

    3. Many clinical subtypes:

          a.   Superficial: scaly erythematous macule or patch.

          b.   Nodular: pearly, translucent papule, or nodule with overlying telangiectasia.

          c.   Pigmented: may resemble a melanoma clinically (black macule or papule). Usually in patients with brown eyes, rare in patients with blue eyes. Very common type in Asians and Hispanics.

          d.   Morphea-like: white scar-like plaque with indurated feel.

          e.   Fibroepithelioma of Pinkus: BCC that commonly occurs as a pink papule on the back but its clinical appearance is variable. Specific unique histologic appearance needed to confirm diagnosis.

    4. Many histologic subtypes.

          a.   Superficial.

          b.   Nodular.

    c. Infiltrative.

    d. Adenoid.

    e. Micronodular.

    f. Adamantinoid.

    g. Morphea-like.

    h. Basosquamous cell (metatypical).

    i. Fibroepithelioma of Pinkus.

> Aggressive histologic subtypes of basal cell carcinoma include infiltrative, adenoid, micronodular, adamantinoid, morphea-like, and basosquamous cell carcinoma.

5. BCCs slowly enlarge and can ulcerate ("rodent ulcer").

    a. 1/2 of deaths that occur from a BCC result from direct extension into a vital structure, such as the carotid artery. Usually these BCCs are very large and have been present for many years.

    b. Metastasis is rare (estimated to be .0028–.55% of BCCs).[1]

6. Some syndromes associated with multiple BCCs.

    a. Nevoid Basal Cell Carcinoma (Gorlin) Syndrome – associated with palmar pits, odontogenic keratocytis, osseous skull anomalies.

    b. Basex Dupre Christol Syndrome – associated with follicular atrophoderma, hypohidrosis, and hypertrichosis.

    c. Linear Unilateral BCC Syndrome – associated with comedones of birth.

7. Treatment: curettage (Figure 4.1) followed by electrocoagulation (C&E), excision, Mohs micrographic surgery, radiation, imiquimod cream, 5-FU, PDT, vismodegib (Erivedge®).

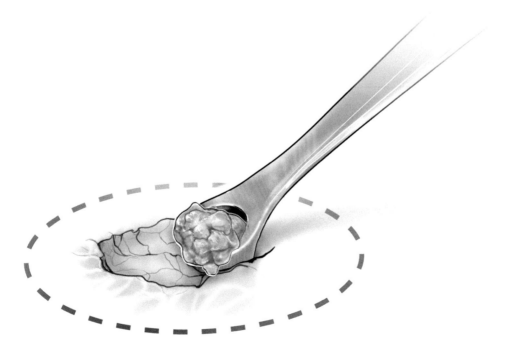

FIGURE 4.1 Curettage of basal or squamous cell carcinoma. Tumor often extends below the surface of visible tumor.

D. Melanoma
   1. Classically appears as a multi-colored black macule/patch that has an irregular border.
      a. Causes the majority of skin cancer deaths.
      b. Metastasizes through lymphatic and hematogenous spread.
   2. About half will develop in pre-existing precursor lesions, such as dysplastic nevi, while about half will develop *de novo.*
      a. ABCDE criterion for identifying a melanoma: Asymmetry, Border irregularity, Color variegation, Diameter large (>6 mm), Evolving (changing) lesion.
      b. Incidence of melanoma has increased, but may be due to better screening methods.
   3. Is commonly believed that sun exposure plays an important role in the causation of melanomas.[4] However, the true significance of sun exposure has been questioned as other factors, such as genetic defects, are discovered.
   4. Melanoma types
      a. In-situ melanoma
         i. Atypical melanocytes and nests are confined to the epidermis and may extend down, the external root sheath around the upper hair follicle.

            There are two types of in-situ melanoma: lentigo maligna type and non-lentigo maligna type.

         ii. There are two types of in-situ melanoma (a.) lentigo maligna type and (b.) non-lentigo maligna type (Table 4.1).
            a) In-situ melanoma lentigo maligna type is common in older people with sun-damaged skin. It appears as a large tan to brown macule or patch with an irregular border on the face or scalp that slowly expands laterally over many years. This lateral expansion when it is histologically confined to the epidermis is known as the horizontal growth phase. When it histologically expands vertically and invades the dermis (the vertical growth phase), it becomes a lentigo maligna melanoma.
            b) In-situ melanoma non-lentigo maligna type is found in young- to middle-aged adults on any skin area but commonly on the trunk and extremities. It is sometimes associated with a nevus. Like an in-situ melanoma lentigo maligna type, single atypical melanocytes and nests are confined to the epidermis and external root sheath. As the melanoma cells histologically expand horizontally and vertically it evolves into a superficial spreading melanoma or a nodular melanoma.

TABLE 4.1

Comparison of Noninvasive Melanomas. Melanoma In Situ (MIS) – Non-Lentigo Maligna Type and Melanoma In Situ – Lentigo Maligna Type

	MIS Non-Lentigo Maligna Type	MIS Lentigo Maligna Type
Surface	Flat or slightly elevated	Flat
Border	Round or slightly irregular	Irregular
Size	Small	Large
Color	Dark brown/black	Brown
Common Locations	Trunk, extremities	Face, scalp
Progression	Unpredictable	Very slow
Tumor Cells	Pagetoid	Spindled

TABLE 4.2

Comparison of Invasive Melanomas. Lentigo Maligna Melanoma (LMM), Superficial Spreading Melanoma (SSM), and Nodular Melanoma (NM)

	LMM	SSM	NM
Surface	Flat	Slightly raised	Nodular
Border	Very irregular	Irregular	Regular
Size	Large (several cm)	Medium (1–5 cm)	Small (<1 cm)
Color	Brown	Variegated	Black
Common Locations	Head, neck, scalp	Leg and upper back	Any
Progression	Very slow	Intermediate	Fast
Tumor Cells	Spindled	Pagetoid	Pagetoid

   b. Lentigo maligna melanoma (LMM) (see Table 4.2).
       i.   Progresses slowly over many years as a lentigo maligna (in- situ melanoma lentigo maligna type) but then develops a vertical growth phase where melanoma cells invade the dermis.
       ii. Occurs on face or heavily sun-damaged skin elsewhere.
       iii. Usually large (>1–2 cm), flat, hyperpigmented lesion with very irregular border (sometimes likened to the shoreline of Maine).
   c. Superficial spreading melanoma (SSM) (see Table 4.1)
       i.   Begins as an in-situ melanoma non-lentigo maligna type that initially appears as smooth macule. With horizontal and/or radial growth becomes a larger macule, patch, or plaque.
       ii. With expansion, the atypical melanocytic cells invade the dermis. At that point the in-situ melanoma becomes a superficial spreading melanoma and appears as a papule or plaque.
       iii. No preference for sun-damaged skin (unlike lentigo maligna).
       iv. Often occurs on the upper back for both sexes and on the legs of women.
       v.   When a vertical growth phase develops, a papule or nodule sometimes appears within the pigmented patch or plaque. This papule or nodule becomes a nodular melanoma within a superficial spreading melanoma.
   d. Nodular melanoma (NM) (see Table 4.1).
       i.   Smooth, dome-shaped black, papular or nodular lesion that can ulcerate (Figure 2.3E). Ulceration is considered a poor prognostic sign.
       ii. May be associated with a superficial spreading melanoma but often appears *de novo* without a horizontal or radial growth phase.
       iii. Accounts for 15% of all melanomas. Usually occurs on the scalp, trunk, and extremities but not the face.
   e. Acral lentiginous melanoma.
       i.   Most common melanoma in Africans, dark-skinned Hispanics and Asians.
       ii. Involves the non-hair bearing glabrous skin of the palms and soles.
       iii. May involve the nail unit most commonly as subungual pigmentation. Brown/black discoloration of the proximal nail fold suggests invasive melanoma. This pigmentation on the nail fold was described by Hutchinson and is often mistakenly referred to as "Hutchinson's sign". The Hutchinson sign is only properly applied to interstitial keratitis and a dull red corneal discoloration associated with congenital syphilis.[5]

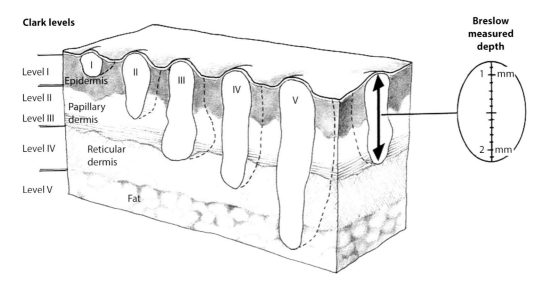

FIGURE 4.2 Comparison of Clark levels and Breslow measured depth to determine skin penetration of melanoma. Clark levels are less used today because they are more subjective than the Breslow measured depth. (Reproduced with permission from Bennett RG, *Fundamentals of Cutaneous Surgery*, C.V. Mosby, St. Louis, 1988.)

    f.   Amelanotic melanoma.
        i.   Rarest form of melanoma. Difficult to spot clinically.
        ii.   Melanoma that lacks pigment: flesh colored, pink or red papule, or nodule.
        iii.   Although usually appears as a nodular melanoma that lacks pigment, lentigo maligna melanomas may also be amelanotic.
        iv.   Typical variant that is seen in albinos.
  5. Melanoma staging.
    a.   Clark Levels[6] (see Figure 4.2).
        i.   Level I: in-situ melanoma.
        ii.   Level II: tumor in the papillary dermis.
        iii.   Level III: tumor abuts the reticular dermis.
        iv.   Level IV: tumor into the reticular dermis.
        v.   Level V: tumor into the subcutaneous fat.
    b.   Breslow measured depth (Figure 4.2).
        i.   <1 mm thickness considered to be superficial and very low risk for metastases.
        ii.   1 mm or greater thickness lesions more likely to metastasize.
    c.   American Joint Committee on Cancer (AJCC) staging classification[7] (see Table 4.3 and Figure 4.3):
        i.   Note that T1- T4, the tumor thickness category is based on pathologically measured depth of melanoma invasion from the top of the granular cell layer to the base of the tumor as defined by Breslow (see Figure 4.2). Breslow depth is considered to be the strongest predictor of survival.
        ii.   As shown in Figure 4.3, the pathologic tumor classification (T) is based on both tumor depth and presence or absence of ulceration.

TABLE 4.3

The Tumor Node Metastasis (TNM) Classification for Melanomas.[*]

	Tis	T1a	T1b	T2a	T2b	T3a	T3b	T4a	T4b	Any T
N0[a]/M0[b]	0	IA	IB[c]	IB	IIA	IIA	IIB	IIB	IIC	
≥ N1/M0										III
Any N/M1										IV

[*] The Roman numerals with or without capital letters refer to the stages.
[a] No regional clinical tumor containing nodes or in transit metastases detected.
[b] No clinical tumor metastasis detected beyond regional site in nodes, skin, lung, viscera, CNS.
[c] Note that for each tumor depth category (T), the clinical and pathologic staging is the same except for T1b. The pathologic staging occurs after sentinel node biopsy. If sentinel node contains no tumor, IB changes to IA.

a) Tis is melanoma in situ. Note that Tis has no depth measurement because tumor cells are confined to the epidermis. Note that whether Tis is ulcerated or not does not change its T classification. Ulceration with Tis is considered to be due to trauma rather than tumor growth, but this is somewhat arbitrary.

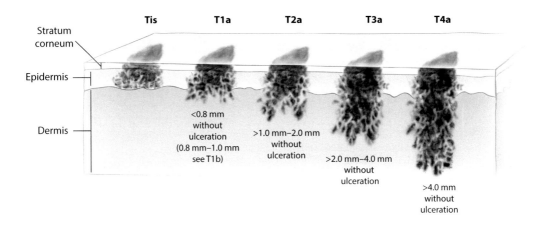

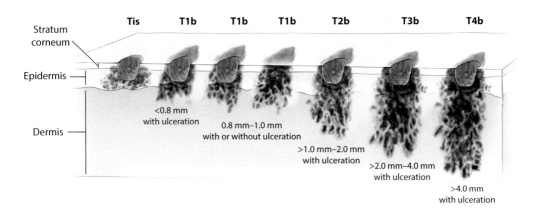

FIGURE 4.3   Histopathologic "T" classification of melanoma based on depth and presence or absence of ulceration. Top: "T" classification without ulceration. Bottom: "T" classification with ulceration. Note that Tis (in situ) is Tis with or without ulceration and tumors 0.8–1 mm with or without ulceration are considered T1b.

  b) Tumor depth is measured from the top of the epidermal granular layer to the lowest level of tumor cells below the epidermis. There are four tumor depth categories (T1-T4).

  c) Note that tumors 0.8–1 mm are considered T1b with or without ulceration.

 iii. Knowing the tumor pathologic T classification and the presence or absence of tumor containing nodes and distant metastases allows one to stage the tumor (Table 4.3). Note the discordance between T classification numbers and letters and stage numbers and letters. Any T tumor with local nodes and no metastases present would be stage III.

 iv. Clark levels are no longer used in this staging classification.

 v. Great weight is given to ulceration of melanoma at any T level except Tis.

 vi. Number of mitosis per mm^2 was considered to be important prognostically but has been abandoned in the most recent 2017 AJCC staging classification.[7]

d. Sentinel lymph node biopsy (SLNB).

 i. A sentinel lymph node is the first node into which a tumor migrates via the lymphatic vessels.

 ii. The identification and biopsy of this node is known as a Sentinel Lymph Node Biopsy (SLNB). Identification of the node is done visually after methylene blue dye injection and/or using lymphoscintigraphy after injection of ^{99m}technetium sulfur colloid.

 iii. Usually recommended for individuals with melanomas >1 mm in thickness.

 iv. Helps to identify regional nodal metastases.

 v. Provides prognostic and survival information but disease free and overall percent survival is not increased with SLN excision and subsequent lymph node dissection (excision of all remaining lymph nodes in the area of the sentinel node if the sentinel lymph node contains melanoma cells).

6. Evaluation

a. For melanoma ≤1 mm thickness.

 i. Complete history, review of systems, past medical history, family history, physical exam including examination of all major lymph nodes (cervical, axillary, inguinal).

 ii. Blood tests: CBC, LDH, LFT.

 iii. Radiologic: CXR.

b. For melanoma ≥1.01 mm thickness.

 i. Complete history, review of systems, past medical history, family history, physical exam including examination of all major lymph nodes – cervical, axillary, inguinal.

 ii. Blood tests: CBC, LDH, LFT.

 iii. Radiologic: CXR, possible PET/CT scan.[8]

 iv. Ophthalmologic exam.

 v. Gynecological examination for women.

7. Treatment

a. Imiquimod cream: used for lentigo maligna (not FDA approved).

b. Radiotherapy: may be useful for lentigo maligna or lentigo maligna melanoma.

c. Excision (recommended excision margins based on Breslow thickness of tumor).

 i. Melanoma in-situ: 0.5 cm margins.

 ii. Melanoma ≤1.0 mm thick: 1 cm margins.

       iii. Melanoma ≤2.0 mm thick: 1–2 cm margins.

       iv. Melanoma >2.0 mm thick: 2 cm margins.

    d. Mohs micrographic surgery using either frozen sections with or without immunostains (Mart-1 or Mel-A), or permanent sections ("slow Mohs").[9] Useful for in-situ melanoma (lentigo and non-lentigo maligna types) and for superficial melanomas <1 mm thickness.

> Mohs micrographic surgery should be considered for all in-situ melanomas especially where tissue preservation is important, e.g., face.

8. Adjuvant therapy.

    a. Consider in patients with positive nodes, or node-negative melanoma that is 4 mm thick, ulcerated or Clark level IV or V.

    b. Interferon-alpha (IFN-α). High-dose IFN-α can increase disease-free survival and possibly overall survival.

    c. Chemotherapy. Dacarbazine (DTIC).

    d. Targeted Therapy. BRAF inhibitor (vemurafenib [Zelboraf®] and dabrafenib [Tafinlar®]) ± MEK inhibitor (trametinib [Mekinist®]).

    e. Immunotherapy. PD-1 (Programmed death-1) inhibitor – pembrolizumab (Keytruda®), nivolumab (Opdivo®), and/or CTLA-4 (cytotoxic T-lymphocyte-associated protein 4) inhibitor – ipilimumab (Yervoy®).

    f. Resection. Prolonged survival can occur in patients treated with surgical resection of limited liver, lung, or brain metastases.

    g. Radiation. Palliative radiation therapy is an option if inoperable brain metastases occur.

E. Extramammary Paget disease (EMPD)

1. Non-healing erythematous patch often misdiagnosed as a fungal infection.

    a. Usually in patients >50 years old.

    b. Affects sites with apocrine glands (vulva, scrotum, inguinal, or axillary regions). When it occurs on the nipple, it is known as Paget's disease.

    c. Two types

       i. Primary EMPD: most common type; only intraepidermal clear (Paget) cells with no underlying or associated carcinoma found.

> Mohs micrographic surgery should be considered for extramammary Paget disease.

       ii. Secondary EMPD: EMPD with underlying cutaneous apocrine carcinoma, EMPD associated with GI malignancy, and EMPD associated with genitourinary cancer.

2. EMPD cells stain with CK7. If EMPD cells stain with CK-20, this may be associated with adenocarcinoma of the rectum, urinary bladder, or cervix.

3. EMPD can invade the dermis and has a high rate of metastasis when such invasion occurs.

4. Obtain serum carcinoembryonic antigen (CEA). A high CEA associated with a large disease burden and decreased survival.

5. Patients may need a sentinel lymph node examination if dermal invasion is present.

6. Treatment: Mohs micrographic surgery, wide local excision (5 cm margins), imiquimod cream, PDT, radiotherapy.

F. Merkel cell carcinoma
   1. Erythematous or violaceous papule.
      a. Very rare. Incidence is two per million.
      b. 95% of cases occur in patients >50 years old.
      c. Associated with Merkel cell polyomavirus (MCV).
   2. Aggressive tumor with dermal and nodal spread.
      a. 30% of cases have regional node involvement and 50% will develop hematogenous spread.
      b. Patients diagnosed with Merkel cell carcinoma should receive a PET/CT scan.
      c. 5 years survival is 64%.
   3. Stains with CK20, chromogranin, and synaptophysin.
   4. Treatment: wide local excision (3 cm margins) with adjuvant radiation treatment, Mohs micrographic surgery, radiation treatment to the region, and associated draining lymph node basin. May consider sentinel lymph node biopsy if no palpable lymph nodes.

G. Dermatofibrosarcoma protuberans (DFSP)
   1. Flesh-colored tumor that can look like a keloid or scar; often multinodular.
      a. Often invades fat and muscle fascia and thus has a high recurrence rate with standard excision.
      b. Can be associated with chromosome 17 and 22 translocations.
      c. 50–60% occur on the trunk.

   Because of its high cure rate, Mohs micrographic surgery should be strongly considered for treatment of dermatofibrosarcoma protuberans.

   2. Stains with CD34. Negative for Factor XIIIa.
   3. Treatment: Mohs micrographic surgery, wide and deep local excision, imatinib (Gleevec®).

H. Sebaceous carcinoma
   1. Rare tumor that often develops on the eyelids where it develops from the glands of Zeis or extraocularly on the face where it develops from sebaceous glands.
      a. When on the eyelids, often misdiagnosed as a chalazion.
      b. Metastatizes 30% of the time in eyelid cases.
      c. May be found with Muir-Torre Syndrome: sebaceous carcinoma/sebaceous adenoma/sebaceomas commonly associated with laryngeal, mammary, or gastrointestinal carcinomas. Genetic testing can be done to establish diagnosis and predict family member susceptibility.
   2. Treatment: Mohs micrographic surgery or wide excision. May consider sentinel lymph node biopsy.

I. Atypical fibroxanthoma (AFX)/pleomorphic dermal sarcoma (PDS)
   1. Typically occurs in elderly individuals on the scalp.
   2. Composed of very atypical fibroblastic cells.
   3. Depth of invasion determines type. If confined to the dermis considered to be AFX. If invades below the dermis considered to be pleomorphic sarcoma.
   4. Treatment: excision, Mohs micrographic surgery, radiation. If a pleomorphic sarcoma, excision should include a 2 cm margin of normal appearing skin and underlying fascia.

J. Microcystic adnexal carcinoma (MAC)
1. Slow-growing flesh-colored plaque or nodule most commonly occurring on the face, especially the upper lip.
a. Local recurrence in 50% of cases treated by standard excision.
b. Perineural invasion is common and may be extensive.
2. Treatment: Mohs micrographic surgery.

Conclusion

Basal cell carcinomas, squamous cell carcinomas, and melanomas are the three most common types of skin cancers and are associated with excessive sun exposure. Many other rare skin cancer types exist. Skin cancer cure rate and prognosis are improved by early detection and adequate treatment. Patients with skin cancers need semiannual or annual skin examinations to detect recurrent or new skin cancers.

REFERENCES

1. James WD, Berger TG, Elston DM. Andrews' Diseases of the Skin: Clinical Dermatology, 10th Edition. Saunders, Canada, 2006.
2. Kauvar ANB, Arpey CJ. et al. Consensus for Nonmelanoma Skin Cancer Treatment, Part II: Squamous Cell Carcinoma, Including a Cost Analysis of Treatment Methods. Dermatol Surg 2015; 41(11): 1214–1240.
3. Weinberg A, Ogle CA, Shim EK. Metastatic Squamous Cell Carcinoma: An Update. Dermatol Surg 2006; 33(8): 885–899.
4. Ivry GB, Ogle CA, Shim EK. Role of Sun Exposure in Melanoma. Dermatol Surg 2006; 32(4): 481–492.
5. Dorland's Illustrated Medical Dictionary, 26th Edition. W.B. Sanders Company, Philadelphia, 1985; p. 1203.
6. McKee PH, Calonje E, Granter SR. Pathology of the Skin, 3rd Edition. Mosby, Philadelphia, 2005.
7. Gershenwald JE, Scolyer RA, Hess KR et al. Melanoma of the skin. In: AJCC Cancer Staging Manual. 8th Edition (Amin MB, Edge S, Greene F et al., editors). Springer, Switzerland, 2017; 563–585.
8. Robinson JK, Hanke CW, Sengelmann RD, Siegel DM, eds. Surgery of the Skin: Procedural Dermatology. Elsevier Mosby, Philadelphia, 2005.
9. Bhardwaj SS, Tope WD, Lee PK. Mohs Micrographic Surgery for Lentigo Maligna and Lentigo Maligna Melanoma Using Mel-5 Immunostaining: University of Minnesota Experience. Dermatol Surg 2006; 32(5): 690–696.

5

Skin Biopsy Techniques

Silvina Pugliese, Tanya Nino, and Abel Torres

Introduction

A skin biopsy is a routine procedure in dermatology. It is used to obtain cutaneous tissue that is examined histologically to diagnose benign and malignant lesions, confirm a cutaneous diagnosis, and identify unusual diseases.[1–4]

I. Preparation

    A. Most skin biopsies are clean procedures, and the area is usually prepped (swabbed) preoperatively with an alcohol swab or other antiseptic agent.

    B. For excisional and some incisional biopsies, the area can be prepped and then draped with a sterile towel to create a sterile field.

    C. The area to be biopsied is circled with a surgical marking pen such as one using gentian violet.

    D. It is a good idea to photograph the lesion to be biopsied so that its location can be easily determined in the future. The patient's cell phone, if available, is a good way to obtain a photograph as this is HIPAA (Health Insurance Portability and Accountability Act of 1996) compliant.

II. Anesthesia

    A. Lidocaine (1%) is the most common local anesthetic used, with or without epinephrine (up to 1:100,000).

    B. Normal saline or diphenhydramine (Benadryl®) may be used for lidocaine-allergic patients. Preservative-free anesthetic solutions are also available such as preservative-free lidocaine (Xylocaine), mepivacaine (Carbocaine®), or bupivacaine (Marcaine®). Usually when the patient states they are allergic to local anesthetics, it is the preservatives he/she is allergic to.

    C. Pearls to minimize the pain from local anesthesia:

        1. Inject very slowly.

        2. Use a small gauge needle (30G is often used).

        3. Use a small syringe (1 or 3 mL) to minimize injection pressures.

        4. Pinch, pat, or press the skin adjacent to the biopsy site prior to injection to provide a distraction. A cool spray like liquid nitrogen can also be used immediately before the biopsy.

> Of all strategies to minimize pain from local anesthesia, very slow injection is most reliable.

5. If it is necessary to re-anesthesize the region, re-enter the skin through an area that has already been anesthetized.

6. An acidic solution causes more pain during injection than a slightly basic solution. Much of the pain of local anesthesia is due to the acidity of an anesthetic solution that contains epinephrine. When possible, use sodium bicarbonate to buffer an epinephrine containing anesthetic solution to above a neutral pH. This can be done by adding one part 8.4% sodium bicarbonate ($NaHCO_3$) to ten parts lidocaine with epinephrine. The addition of $NaHCO_3$ raises the pH of the epinephrine containing anesthetic solution into the basic range. Unfortunately, the local anesthetic with its pH altered by sodium bicarbonate does not have a long shelf life and should be used within a few days.

7. Warm the anesthetic closer to body temperature (37°C) before injection.

D. Topical anesthetic cream, such as EMLA™ (2.5% lidocaine with 2.5% prilocaine), may be used.

1. Generally does not penetrate intact skin.

2. Anatomic locations where topical anesthetic cream application works well include the eyelids, mucosal surfaces (vermillion of lips), and genitalia. These are areas where the dermis is very thin. Anesthesia in these areas is achieved with a 5–10 minutes application, even without overlying semiocclusive bandages.

3. Anatomic locations where topical anesthetic application does not work well include all areas where the dermis is thick, such as the trunk, extremities, and face (except eyelids). If used in these areas need to apply overlying semiocclusive dressing for 30–45 minutes.

4. Although used commonly prior to local anesthetic injection or vaccination injection in the pediatric population, it probably will not work well.

5. Covering the anesthetic cream with an occlusive dressing (e.g., Tegaderm™) helps the anesthetic penetrate the skin.

III. Skin Biopsy Types (Table 5.1)

A. Scissors biopsy

1. Indications:
   a. Pedunculated lesions (e.g., skin tags) (see Figure 3.3A and B)
2. Technique:
   a. Pull the lesion away from the skin using forceps, but do not crush the tissue.
   b. Snip the base of the lesion with small scissors, such as iris, Gradle, or tenotomy scissors.

B. Shave (nearly horizontal) biopsy

1. Types:
   a. Superficial shave: includes predominantly epidermis and superficial (papillary) dermis.

TABLE 5.1

Comparison of Shave Biopsy, Punch Biopsy, Incisional Biopsy, and Excisional Biopsy

	Shave Biopsy	**Punch Biopsy**	**Incisional Biopsy**	**Excisional Biopsy**
Instrument	Scalpel or razor blade	Skin punch	Scalpel blade	Scalpel blade
Removal	Partial or complete	Partial or complete	Partial	Complete
Orientation	Almost horizontal	Vertical	Vertical	Vertical
Sutured	No	Yes	Yes	Yes
Depth	Superficial	Deep	Deep	Deep

(a)   (b)

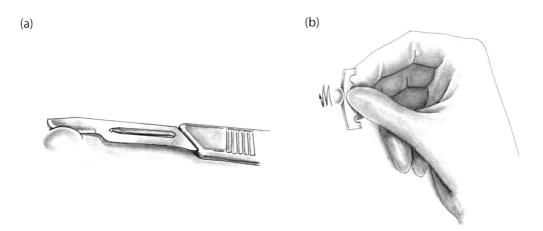

FIGURE 5.1   Horizontal (shave) biopsy using (A) #15 blade or (B) Razor blade. (Reproduced with permission from Bennett R.G., *Fundamentals of Cutaneous Surgery*, C.V. Mosby, St. Louis, 1988.)

   b.   Deep shave/saucerization: includes epidermis and mid-dermis.
2. Indications:
   a.   Superficial: exophytic lesions.
   b.   Saucerization: gaining popularity in the removal of pigmented lesions suspected of being melanoma, but must make sure it is deep enough to allow for depth evaluation of any microscopic dermal penetration.
3. Technique:
   a.   After the skin is anesthetized, a #15 scalpel blade (Figure 5.1A) or a flexible razor blade (Figure 5.1B) can be used to remove the lesion.
   b.   For superficial shave biopsies, the scalpel is held like a pencil and its blade is moved in a smooth back and forth motion parallel to the skin surface.
   c.   For saucerization shave biopsies, a deep biopsy is obtained by adjusting the angle of the blade to "scoop" out the desired skin. Non-sterile flexible razor blades (Figure 5.1B) provide increased control in this regard, allowing the user to increase concavity by flexing the sides of the blade by compressing the blade with the thumb and index fingers holding the blade. Sterile flexible razor-type blades (e.g., Derma Blade [Medex]) are also available with grips on either side for ease of handling.
4. Considerations:
   a.   The immediate wheal produced by the injection of local anesthesia can be useful in lifting the lesion away from the surrounding skin, thus facilitating its removal. However, if the shave biopsy is performed with this wheal, it may produce a dell in the skin after the resultant wound is healed.

   > Be careful performing a shave biopsy on a lesion elevated by local anesthetic solution – a subsequent dell-shaped scar may result.

   b.   No sutures are necessary as the wound heals by second intention.
C. Punch biopsy
1. Indications:
   a.   Skin condition necessitating evaluation of the dermis and/or subcutaneous fat.
   b.   Tissue culture for deep fungal infection.

Skin punch

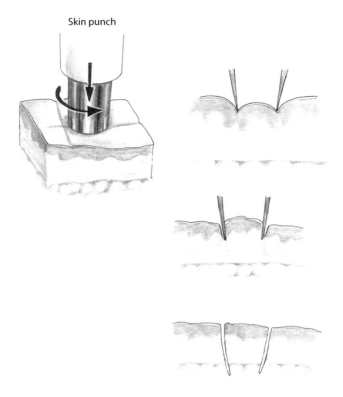

FIGURE 5.2   (A and B) Punch biopsy: Motion of a skin punch to take a cone-shaped biopsy. Note that as it penetrates the skin, the punch is not rotated back and forth but rotated in one direction. (Reproduced with permission from Bennett R.G., *Fundamentals of Cutaneous Surgery*, C.V. Mosby, St. Louis, 1988.)

2. Technique:
   a. After the skin is anesthetized, a trephine (skin punch) is pushed through the skin with a turning and downward movement. Avoid back-and-forth twisting as this usually does not result in a clean edge (Figure 5.2).
   b. The specimen should be lifted gently, using forceps to grip one tissue edge gingerly and scissors to cut the punch biopsy base, ensuring that the entirety of the sample is removed without tissue crimping.
   c. After the specimen is removed, interrupted sutures may be placed to close the wound and for hemostasis.
3. Considerations:
   a. A skin punch is an instrument with a sharp cutting edge at the end of a cylindrical-shaped head. It is available in sizes ranging from less than 0.5 mm to 10 mm. The skin punch size chosen is contingent on a number of variables, including the lesion size, lesion location, and the most likely location of the pathology for which one is performing the biopsy. Most punch biopsies are done with a 3 mm or 4 mm skin punch.
   b. If the subcutaneous fat is the area of interest, a deep biopsy should be obtained. Often, this necessitates the use of two consecutive, or "stacked", punch biopsies. For example, an 8 mm punch biopsy may be utilized to enter the skin, with a 4 mm punch biopsy to follow. A punch biopsy may not be as useful when the fat is inflamed, as it may fall away from the specimen as it is lifted from the biopsy site.

    c. Stretching the skin perpendicular to relaxed skin tension lines prior to punch incision will often result in an elliptical wound which will close with minimal standing cones (dog ears).

    d. Squeezing the punch biopsy specimen too firmly between the forceps tips can cause "crush" artifact, which shreds the tissue and makes pathologic examination difficult. Thus, be careful when lifting the specimen from its base.

> Stretching the skin perpendicular to the skin tension lines will often produce an elliptical wound when using a round skin punch.

D. Incisional and excisional biopsies

    1. Definitions: (Figure 5.3)

        a. Incisional biopsy: removal of part of a lesion.

        b. Excisional biopsy: removal of an entire lesion.

    2. Indications:

        a. Incisional biopsies can be used to assess pathology within the fat as well as to sample a portion of a very large tumor.

        b. Excisional biopsies can be used to clinically remove small lesions. Excisional biopsies for melanomas minimize sampling error and render a more accurate depth of invasion necessary or accurate staging (see Table 4.2).

IV. Hemostasis Technique

A. Physical methods include pressure and bandages. Pressure may need to be applied for 15–20 minutes without peeking.

B. Chemical methods include aluminum chloride (30% $AlCl_3$ hydrated) or 20% aluminum chloride hexahydrate (Drysol™), 20% ferric subsulfate solution (Monsel's solution), and silver nitrate sticks (75% silver nitrate and 25% potassium nitrate).

C. Electrical methods include electrocautery or high-frequency electrosurgery (such as electrodesiccation and electrocoagulation).

D. Suturing methods include percutaneous stitches. Rarely, if a small artery is bleeding it may need to be ligated with an absorbable suture.

V. Aftercare

A. Keep area moist with an antibacterial ointment or vaseline to promote wound healing.

B. Wash with soap and water. Hydrogen peroxide (3%) may also be used.

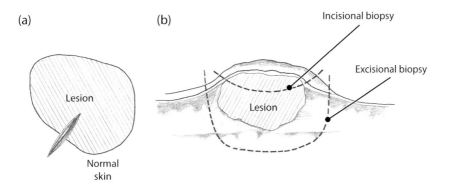

FIGURE 5.3 (A) Incisional biopsy that includes a portion of the lesion and a portion of normal skin that may be important to show histologically the transition between the lesion and the normal skin. (B) Comparison of excisional biopsy and incisional biopsy. (Reproduced with permission from Bennett R.G., *Fundamentals of Cutaneous Surgery*, C.V. Mosby, St. Louis, 1988.)

C. Keep wound covered with a bandage until healed.

D. Note that an antibiotic ointment (especially Neomycin or Polysporin ointment) may cause an allergic contact dermatitis. If this occurs, have patient use plain vaseline.

Conclusion

Although a skin biopsy is a minor procedure, selection of the best technique for a given lesion requires some knowledge of dermatology and the limits of each method.

REFERENCES

1. Affleck AG, Colver G. Skin biopsy techniques. In: Surgery of the Skin: Procedural Dermatology (Robinson JK, Hanke CW, Siegel DM, Fratila A, editors). Elsevier, New York, NY, 2010.

2. James WD, Berger TG, Elston DM. Dermatologic surgery. In: Andrews' Diseases of the Skin: Clinical Dermatology. 11th Edition. Elsevier, New York, NY, 2011.

3. High WA, Tomasini CF, Argenziano G, Zalaudek I. Basic principles of dermatology. In: Dermatology. 3rd Edition (Bolognia JL, Jorizzo JL, Schaffer JV, editors). Elsevier, New York, NY, 2012.

4. Marks JG, Miller JJ. Dermatologic therapy and procedures. In: Lookingbill & Marks' Principles of Dermatology. 4th Edition. Elsevier, New York, NY, 2006.

Section II

Dermatologic Surgery Basics

6

Wound Healing

Teresa Soriano

Introduction

Surgical wounds typically heal by following a sequence of three overlapping physiological stages: inflammation, proliferation, and remodeling.[1] Normal wound healing can be prolonged in individuals with certain diseases such as diabetes and vascular insufficiencies as well as other factors such as malnutrition, smoking, prior radiation, and infection.

I. Wound Healing Sequence for a Typical Sutured Wound (Figure 6.1)
  A. Hemostasis (0–15 minutes)
    1. Vasoconstriction and clot formation.
    2. Clotting cascade results in fibrin formation.[2–4]
      a. Platelet aggregation and degranulation activates coagulation cascade.
      b. Thrombin stimulated cleavage of fibrinogen to fibrin.
      c. Fibrin monomers crosslinked by factor XIIIa.
      d. Fibrin binds to platelets to form a clot.
  B. Inflammatory phase (days 1–3)
    1. Capillary vasodilation, increased vascular permeability, and cellular influx with recruitment.
    2. Early phase.
      a. Neutrophil recruitment into the wound.[5,6]
        i. Degranulated platelets, activated complement pathway, and bacterial by-products recruit neutrophils to injured tissue.
        ii. Peak neutrophil numbers at 24–48 hours.
        iii. Remove cellular debris and bacteria.
        iv. Release antimicrobial substances (cationic peptides and eicosanoids).
        v. Release proteinases (elastase, cathepsin G, urokinase-type plasminogen activator).
        vi. Produce cytokines such as interleukin-1 alpha (IL-1α), IL-1β, IL-6, tumor necrosis factor alpha (TNF-α) that amplify inflammatory response.
        vii. Stimulate vascular endothelial growth factor (VEGF) and IL-8 for optimal wound healing.
    3. Late phase.
      a. Monocytes populate wound and transform into macrophages.[5–7]
        i. Peak numbers at 48–72 hours and remain for weeks.
        ii. Macrophages produce potent cytokines and growth factors such as tumor growth factor beta (TGF-β), tumor growth factor alpha (TGF-α), basic fibroblast growth factor (FGF), platelet-derived growth factor (PDGF), and VEGF.
        iii. Macrophages also function as antigen presenting cells to provide host defense and phagocytose apoptotic cells.

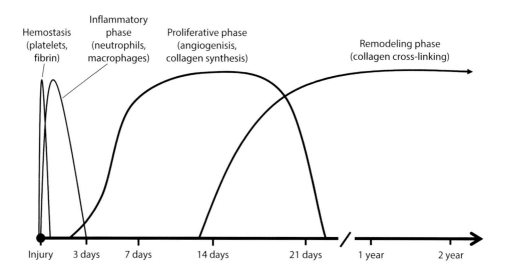

FIGURE 6.1   Hemostasis and three wound healing phases for a typical sutured wound.

C. Proliferative phase (2 days–3 weeks)

1. Secretion of growth factors, synthesis of collagen III, extracellular matrix formed, and beginning of angiogenesis.[5,7]

2. Epidermization.

    a. Basal cell proliferation and/or epidermal cell migration below the fibrin clot.

    b. Keratinocytes at wound edges and epithelial stem cells from hair follicles and sweat glands participate in re-epithelialization.

    c. In sutured wounds, process is completed in as early as 48 hours.

    d. Wounds healing by secondary intention have prolonged re-epidermization process due to increased distance necessary for epidermal migration.

    e. Growth factors and cytokines such as TGF-β, FGF-2, nerve growth factor (NGF), and human growth factor (HGF) contribute to epidermal migration.

    f. Matrix metalloproteinases (MMPs) such as MMP-1 also play a role in keratinocyte migration.

3. Granulation tissue formation.

    a. Angiogenesis. Restoration of vascular network across wound involves cellular, molecular, and humoral mechanisms.

    b. Low oxygen tension and lactic acid help stimulate endothelial cell proliferation.

    c. Growth factors, such as VEGF, FGF, angiopoeitin, and TGF-β are important for angiogenesis.[8,9]

    d. Fibrous tissue formation.

        i. Replaces fibrin-based wound matrix.

        ii. High density of fibroblasts, macrophages, granulocytes, and loosely organized collagen bundles.

            a) Fibroblasts produce collagen and extracellular matrix substances such as fibronectin, glycosaminoglycans, proteoglycans, and hyaluronic acid.

        b) Collagen production begins 3–5 days after injury.

        c) In early wound healing, collagen III is deposited and comprises approximately 30% of dermal collagen.

        d) Normal skin has 80–90% collagen type I and 10–20% collagen type III.

        e) Collagen production stimulated by growth factors including PDGF, TGF-β, and EGF.

D. Remodeling phase (2 weeks–2 years)[5]

   1. Wound contraction and relaxation, decreased erythema and induration, and increased wound strength.

   2. Wound contraction starts 4–5 days after injury and continues for approximately 2 weeks.

      a. PDGF and TGF-β contribute to fibroblast phenotypic transformation to myofibroblasts.

      b. Myofibroblasts have contractile properties due to increased actin-like filaments.

> Wound contraction may result in distortion (known as contracture) of a nearby structure such as an eyelid or lip.

   3. Net collagen production by fibroblasts increases until approximately day 21.

   4. Interferon alpha (IFNα) and TNF-α trigger decrease collagen production.

   5. MMPs contribute to extracellular matrix remodeling.

   6. New collagen formation.

      a. Increased proportion of type I collagen relative to type III collagen.

      b. Increased diameter and rearrangement of collagen fibrils.

   7. Crosslinking of collagen fibrils.

      a. Leads to increased wound breaking and tensile strength.

   8. Wound strength does not achieve 100% of previous strength prior to wounding.

      a. At 3 weeks, tensile wound strength is approximately 20% of baseline.

      b. At 6–12 months, tensile wound strength is approximately 80% of baseline.

   9. Mature wound is less vascular and less cellular.

      a. Fibroblast numbers decrease.

      b. Antiangiogenic factors, like thrombospondin, contribute to decreased vascularity.

      c. Skin epithelial appendages are lacking in scar tissue.

II. Important Wound Healing Terms

A. Contraction versus contracture: contracture is the distortion of surrounding tissue caused by wound contraction. Oftentimes the distortion is of a free edge, e.g., eyelid, alar rim. Wound contraction occurs in wounds extending through the dermis, i.e., a full thickness wound.

B. Epidermization (or re-epidermization) versus epithelialization (or re-epithelialization): epidermization occurs when the epidermis reforms from the wounds edges only. The new epidermis is flat and devoid of dermal pupillae, hair follicles, or sweat ducts. Epithelialization (or re-epithelialization) occurs when the epidermis reforms from both the wound edges and the underlying hair follicles and sweat ducts. Thus, a functioning epithelium is formed not only with epidermis but also with hair follicles and sweat ducts.

III. Types of Wound Healing

A. First versus second versus third intention

   1. First intention wound healing refers to a wound that heals by immediate suturing.

   2. Second intention wound healing refers to a wound that is not sutured but allowed to heal naturally through the processes of granulation, contraction, and re-epidermization (Figure 6.2).

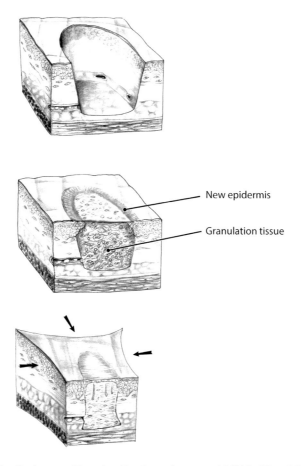

FIGURE 6.2   Wound healing by second intention. Top: Large deep wound. Middle: Wound filled with granulation tissue. Granulation tissue contraction drawing wound edges together. New epidermis beginning to grow over granulation tissue. Bottom: Wound completely healed by second intention. Note resultant scar (Bottom) is smaller than size of original wound (Top) due to contractile forces (shown by arrows) of granulation tissue. (Reproduced with permission from Bennett RG, *Fundamentals of Cutaneous Surgery*, C.V. Mosby, St. Louis, 1988.)

      3. Tertiary intention wound healing refers to a wound that is allowed to heal naturally for a short period of time (usually 2–3 weeks) by granulation and contraction and then repaired with a skin graft or flap.

  IV. Types of Wounds

      A. Depth and width (Figure 6.3)

          1. Superficial abrasions.

             a. Narrow or wide.

             b. Heal by epidermization from wound edges and from adnexal structures (hair follicules, sweat ducts) in the wound base to produce functional re-epithelialized tissue. In the skin, the functional epithelium includes the epidermis with its adnexal structures (sweat ducts, hair follicles, and sebaceous glands) that course through the epidermis.

             c. If abrasion is very superficial to papillary dermis only, there is no scarring.

             d. If abrasion extends to reticular dermis, noticeable scarring and slight contraction might occur.

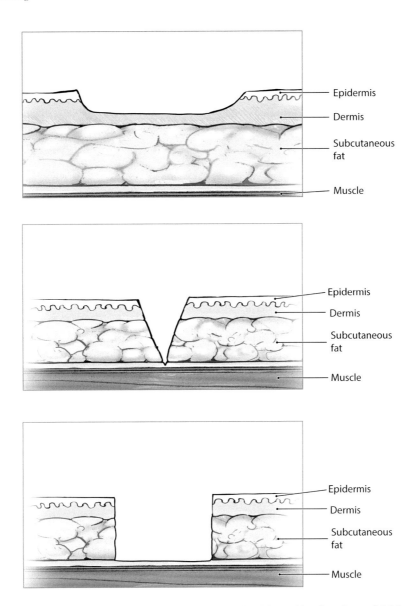

FIGURE 6.3 Different types of wounds. (Top) Superficial wound involving epidermis and superficial dermis. (Middle) Typical incision type wound into subcutaneous tissue. Note retraction of surrounding skin resulting in a gaping wound. (Bottom) A wide and deep wound into subcutaneous tissue. (Modified from Bennett RG, *Fundamentals of Cutaneous Surgery*, C.V. Mosby, St. Louis, 1988.)

2. Narrow deep wound.
   a. Usually sutured.
   b. Heals by granulation (fibroblasts and angiogenesis) and re-epidermization.
3. Wide deep wound.
   a. May be repaired with skin graft or skin flap.
   b. May be allowed to heal by second intention (granulation, contraction, epidermization) (see Figure 6.2).

V. Wound Care for Nonchronic Wounds

   A. Sutured wound

      1. Use ointment, nonstick absorbent dressing, gauze, and paper tape for first 24 hours.

      2. After 24 hours dressing changed and daily thereafter until suture removal.

      3. Wound kept moist until suture removal. For each dressing change, wound is cleaned with hydrogen peroxide, patted dry with gauze, ointment applied, followed by application of nonstick bandage and paper tape.

      4. Patient can get dressing wet after 24 hours.

      5. At time of suture removal, skin tackifier and paper strips are usually applied to reinforce wound strength.

   B. Non-sutured wound. Wound kept moist until healed completely. For abrasions, this takes 1–2 weeks. For deep post-Mohs surgical wounds, the average time for healing is 6 weeks.

      1. First dressing change at 24 hours and daily thereafter until completely healed.

      2. Dressing changes as follows: wound cleansed with hydrogen peroxide or sterile saline, patted dry with gauze, ointment and nonstick absorbent dressing applied, and paper tape on all sides of dressing to maintain moist seal in wound. Although some believe that hydrogen peroxide delays wound healing, from a practical point of view we have not found this to be true with one exception. On the scalp, when deep wounds are almost completely re-epidermized. The hydrogen peroxide, because of its effervescent effect, tends to lift off the poorly adherent new epidermis. If this happens, we usually substitute normal saline to cleanse the wound.

      3. During early wound healing on the leg, a yellow fibrinous exudate may form that is normal. This is left in place.

      4. Exudate may coalesce with the topical ointment to form a white coagulum that can be gently lifted off.

      5. Contact dermatitis can occur at any point in the wound healing process. Usually this is due to an antibiotic ointment. We usually substitute Vaseline to keep the wound moist and prescribe triamcinolone acetonide 0.1% ointment for the red pruritic rash around the open wound.

      6. Signs that the wound is completely healed.

         a. The peroxide no longer bubbles when applied to the wound.

         b. There is no longer drainage on the underside of nonstick bandage.

VI. Risk Factors for Delayed Wound Healing

   A. Smoking

      1. Associated with increased post-operative infection, wound necrosis, and dehiscence.[10,11]

      2. Negative effects on wound healing.

         a. Enhances vasoconstriction leading to surgical site ischemia.

         b. Reduces inflammatory response.

         c. Alters normal collagen metabolism.

         d. Impairs antibacterial wound processes.

   B. Diabetes

      1. Associated with vasculopathy, neuropathy, immunopathy.[12,13]

      2. Impairs fibroblast migration and proliferation, growth factor production, and macrophage function.

   C. Chronic venous insufficiency

      1. Lower extremity wounds particularly at risk for delayed healing.

      2. Chronic periwound edema alters myofibroblast activity and collagen deposition.

    D. Diseases that result in tissue ischemia
        1. Peripheral artery disease.
        2. Vasculitis.
        3. Other disorders associated with microvascular thrombosis.
    E. Malnutrition[14]
        1. Common in elderly, especially with poor diet.
        2. Increases risk for wound infection and delayed wound healing.

> Delayed wound healing occurs in elderly patients with poor nutritional intake.

    F. Prior radiation therapy[15]
        1. Produces fibroplasia that results in decreased vascular supply which impairs normal wound healing.
    G. Infection
        1. Bacterial production of anti-inflammatory mediators inhibit inflammatory phase of wound healing and prevent re-epidermization.
    H. Medications
        1. Examples: systemic retinoids, sirolimus, chemotherapy (variable), systemic steroids.[16,17]

VII. Strategies for non-healing wounds. Chronic wounds where the process of normal wound healing has been arrested at a specific stage of healing.
    A. Measure the wound size on each office visit to document progress or non-progress of wound healing.
    B. Obtain wound culture. If culture shows gram-negative organisms, consider acetic acid solution or silver nitrate solution 0.25–0.5% applied for 5–10 minutes on gauze soaked in solution (Table 10.5).
    C. Clean wound with hydrogen peroxide 3% or sterile normal saline once or twice a day. Hydrogen peroxide has an effervescent effect that helps to debride the wound. As pointed out previously, this effervescent effect may lift off newly formed epidermis on the scalp where it is poorly adherent at first.
    D. Apply antibiotic ointment (Table 9.1).
    E. Keep wound covered and moist with nonstick dressing (e.g., Telfa) and paper tape to make sure wound is sealed to create a moist environment.
    F. May consider special dressings such as synthetic dressings (Table 9.2) or biologic dressings (Table 9.3).
    G. Debridement of necrotic tissue may be considered.
    H. For wounds with hypergranulation tissue, can curette, horizontally excise (shave), or apply silver nitrate 40% on a wooden stick.
    I. To prepare the non-healing wound for closure remove 1–2 mm rim of epidermis and possibly superficial wound base. The wound is then irrigated with a copious amount of sterile saline.
    J. Close the wound either side to side or with a skin flap or skin graft.

Conclusion

Following surgery, wound healing occurs through a cascade of events that begins with hemostasis, then progresses through inflammatory, proliferative, and remodeling stages, and ends with the formation of scar tissue. In normal individuals, this process proceeds in a predictable time period; however, certain conditions such as diabetes, smoking, infection, and prior radiation therapy can delay wound healing. Knowledge of the key elements of acute wound healing will assist in optimal patient selection and perioperative care in cutaneous surgery.

REFERENCES

1. Baum C, Arpey C. Normal Cutaneous Wound Healing: Clinical Correlation With Cellular and Molecular Events. Dermatol Surg 2005; 31: 674–686.
2. Eming SA. Inflammation in Wound Repair: Molecular and Cellular Mechanisms. J Invest Dermatol 2007; 127: 514–525.
3. Blomback B, Hessel B, Hogg D, Therkildsen L. A Two-Step Fibrinogen-Fibrin Transition in Blood Coagulation. Nature 1978; 275: 501–505.
4. Mosesson MW, Siebenlist KR, Meh DA. The Structure and Biological Features of Fibrinogen and Fibrin. Ann N Y Acad Sci 2001; 936: 11–30.
5. Lawrence WT. Physiology of the Acute Wound. Clin Plast Surg 1998; 25: 321–340.
6. Werner S, Grose R. Regulation of Wound Healing by Growth Factors and Cytokines. Physio Rev 2003; 83: 835–870.
7. Singer AJ, Clark RAF. Cutaneous Wound Healing. N Engl J Med 1999; 341: 738–746.
8. Steed D. The Role of Growth Factors in Wound Healing. Surg Clin North Am 1997; 77: 575–586.
9. Li J, Zhang Y-P, Kirsner RS. Angiogenesis in Wound Repair: Angiogenic Growth Factors and the Extracellular Matrix. Microsc Res Tech 2003; 60: 107–114.
10. Silverstein P. Smoking and Wound Healing. Am J Med 2002; 93(1A): 22S–24S.
11. Jensen JA, Goodson WH, Hopf HW et al. Cigarette Smoking Decreases Tissue Oxygen. Arch Surg 1991; 126: 1131–1132.
12. Algenstaedt P, Schaefer C, Biermann T et al. Microvascular Alterations in Diabetic Mice Correlate With Hyperglycemia. Diabetes 2003; 52: 542–549.
13. Carrico TJ, Mehrhof AI, Coehn IK. Biology of Wound Healing. Surg Clin N Am 1984; 64: 921–933.
14. Pollack S. Wound Healing: A Review III. Nutritional Factors Affecting Wound Healing. Dermatol Surg 1979; 5(8): 615–619.
15. Miller SH, Rudolph R. Healing in the Irradiated Wound. Clin Plast Surg 1990; 17: 503–508.
16. Anstead GM. Steroids, Retinoids, and Wound Healing. Adv Wound Care 1998; 11: 227–285.
17. Karukonda SR, Flynn TC, Boh EE et al. The Effects of Drugs on Wound Healing-Part II. Specific Classes of Drugs and Their Effect on Healing Wounds. Int J Dermatol 2000; 64: 986–994.

7

Anatomy

Allison Hanlon

Introduction

A comprehensive knowledge in anatomy is a key foundation for dermatologic surgery. Anatomical study begins with an understanding of the superficial anatomy of the skin – how the skin topography relates to critical deep structures such as nerves and blood vessels. Surface anatomy nomenclature is important to accurately identify the exact procedure location and to localize important structures deep to the superficial anatomical landmarks. Further, surgical planning with respect to anatomic landmarks and structures is essential for optimal surgical outcomes.[1,2]

I. Head and Neck
  A. The cosmetic subunits are regions sharing common color, texture, and sebaceous or non-sebaceous skin.
    1. Cosmetic subunits include the forehead, glabella, temple, cheek, chin, eyelids, nose, ear, and neck.
    2. The cosmetic subunits are bordered by several anatomic lines, folds or sulci, including the melolabial crease (between the cheek and upper lip), the nasofacial sulcus (between the nose and cheek), the mental crease (between the chin and lower lip), and the preauricular sulcus (between the ear and preauricular cheek) (Figure 7.1).
  B. In the lateral neck, the underlying sternocleidomastoid muscle divides the neck into two triangles: the anterior cervical triangle and the posterior cervical triangle. The anterior cervical triangle is bounded by the mandible superiorly, by the sternocleidomastoid muscle posteriorly, and by the midline neck anteriorly. The posterior cervical triangle is bounded by the sternocleidomastoid muscle anteriorly, the clavicle inferiorly, and the border of the trapezius muscle posteriorly. These two triangles are important for describing the location of cancer containing nodes.
  C. Maximum skin tension lines (sometimes referred to as relaxed skin tension lines or Langer lines) are lines oriented along the direction of maximum skin tension.
    1. These lines are usually parallel to the wrinkle lines (Figure 7.2).
    2. These lines are usually perpendicular to the underlying superficial muscles.[1]
    3. To achieve an optimal cosmetic result, surgical scar placement is best oriented along the maximum skin tension lines.
  D. Surface anatomy
    1. Nose (Figure 7.3).
    2. Ear (Figure 7.4).

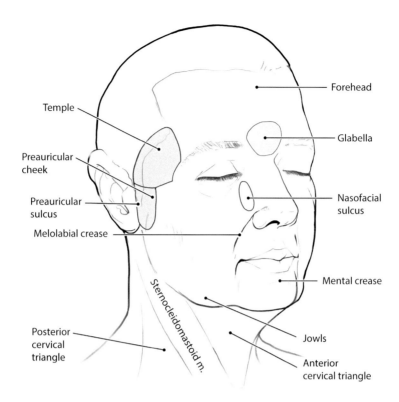

Forehead

Temple

Glabella

Preauricular cheek

Preauricular sulcus

Nasofacial sulcus

Melolabial crease

Sternocleidomastoid m.

Mental crease

Posterior cervical triangle

Jowls

Anterior cervical triangle

FIGURE 7.1   Anatomic lines, creases, and sulci of head and neck.

   E.   Sensory innervation
      1.   Ear (Figure 7.5).
         a.   Cranial nerves VII, IX, and X innervate the concha. Cranial nerve VII also inner-
              vates the posterior earlobe. Cranial nerves IX and X may also contribute to inner-
              vate the lower posterior sulcus.
         b.   The auriculotemporal nerve, a branch of the mandibular division (V_3) of the tri-
              geminal nerve, innervates the superior proximal portion of the posterior helix and
              most of the medial anterior ear above the level of the tragus.
         c.   The great auricular nerve (C_2, C_3) innervates most of the remaining posterior ear,
              the inferior anterior ear below the level of the tragus, and the upper distal half of
              the anterior ear.
         d.   The lesser occipital nerve (mainly C_2) arises superior to the great auricular nerve
              on the anterior side of the sternocleidomastoid muscle. This nerve innervates most
              of the posterior auricular sulcus and the mastoid scalp (not shown separately in
              Figure 7.5).
      2.   Face.
         a.   Trigeminal nerve (cranial nerve V) divides into three branches for sensory innervation of the face (Figure 7.6).
            i.   Ophthalmic division (V_1) divides into the frontal nerve, the lacrimal nerve, and the nasociliary nerve.
               a)   Frontal nerve divides into the supratrochlear nerve and the

On each side of the nose, the external nasal branch of the anterior ethmoidal nerve exits between the nasal bone and nasal cartilage to innervate the tip of the nose. When performing a nerve block of the total nose this nerve is sometimes overlooked.

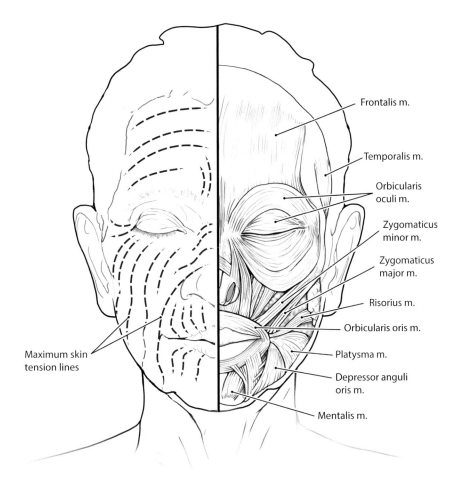

Frontalis m.

Temporalis m.

Orbicularis oculi m.

Zygomaticus minor m.

Zygomaticus major m.

Risorius m.

Orbicularis oris m.

Maximum skin tension lines

Platysma m.

Depressor anguli oris m.

Mentalis m.

FIGURE 7.2 Maximum skin tension lines of the face. Note that these generally are perpendicular to the underlying superficial facial muscles.

supraorbital nerve. The supratrochlear nerve innervates the lower medial forehead. The supraorbital nerve innervates the mid lateral to lateral forehead, frontal scalp, and upper eyelid.

b) The lacrimal nerve innervates the conjunctiva and usually the skin on the lateral corner of the eyelids.

c) The nasociliary nerve divides into the posterior ethmoidal, the anterior ethmoidal, and the infratrochlear nerves. The infratrochlear nerve innervates the upper lateral aspect of the nose and the medial upper and lower eyelids. The anterior ethmoidal nerve divides into an external and an internal nasal branch. The external nasal branch runs inferiorly on the inner surface of the nasal bone, exits between the nasal bone and the lateral nasal cartilage, and supplies the skin on the lower half of the dorsum of the nose.[3]

ii. Maxillary division (V_2) divides into the infraorbital nerve, zygomaticofacial nerve, and zygomaticotemporal nerve.

a) Infraorbital nerve exits from a small foramen in the anterior maxilla and innervates medial cheek, upper lip, nasal sidewall, ala, and lower eyelid.

b) Zygomaticofacial branch exits from a small foramen in the zygomatic bone and innervates the malar eminence.

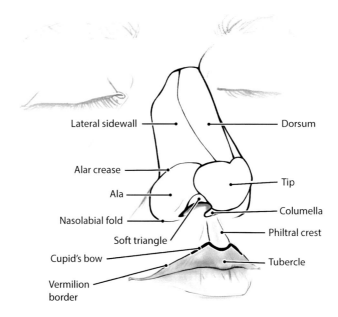

FIGURE 7.3 Nasal subunits.

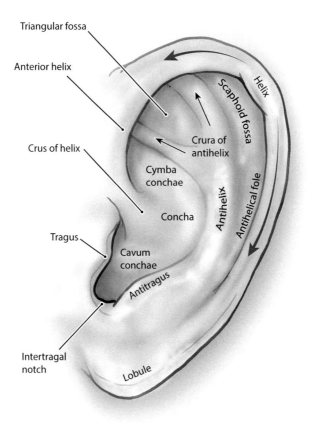

FIGURE 7.4 Subunits of the ear.

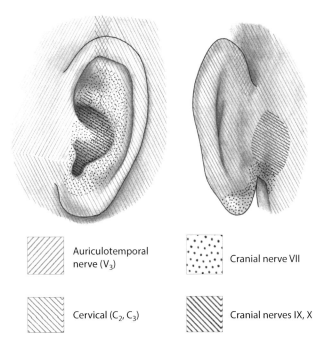

| | Auriculotemporal nerve (V_3) | | Cranial nerve VII |
| | Cervical (C_2, C_3) | | Cranial nerves IX, X |

FIGURE 7.5 Sensory innervation of the anterior and posterior ear. Note that the C_2, C_3 distribution on the sulcus and mastoid scalp is from the lesser occipital nerve. The remainder of the C_2, C_3 distribution is from the great auricular nerve. (Modified from Bennett RG, *Fundamentals of Cutaneous Surgery*, C.V. Mosby, St. Louis, 1988.)

      c) Zygomaticotemporal branch exits at the superior edge of the zygomatic bone and innervates the temple and supratemporal scalp.

    iii. Mandibular branch (V_3) divides into the auriculotemporal nerve, buccal nerve, and inferior alveolar nerve.

      a) Auriculotemporal nerve innervates a portion of the external ear, auditory canal, temple, temporoparietal scalp, temporomandibular joint, and tympanic membrane.

      b) Buccal nerve innervates the cheek, buccal mucosa, and gingiva.

      c) Inferior alveolar nerve innervates the mandibular teeth and continues as the mental nerve to innervate the chin and lower lip. The lingual nerve branches from the inferior alveolar nerve and innervates the anterior two-thirds of the tongue.

F. Motor innervation

  1. Facial nerve (Cranial Nerve VII) innervates the muscles of facial expression (Figure 7.7).

    a. Branches include temporal, zygomatic, buccal, marginal mandibular, and cervical. Note that there is a great anatomic variability and interconnections between the branches. Often two branches come off the facial nerve together, e.g., temporal and zygomatic branches.

      i. Temporal branch innervates frontalis, orbicularis oculi, corrugator supercilii, and procerus muscles.

      ii. Zygomatic branch innervates lower orbicularis oculi, procerus, nasalis, levator anguli oris, and zygomaticus major muscles.

      iii. Buccal branch innervates buccinator, depressor septi nasii, nasalis, orbicularis oris, levator labii superioris, levator anguli oris, zygomaticus major and minor, and risorius muscles. Zygomatic and buccal branches have numerous

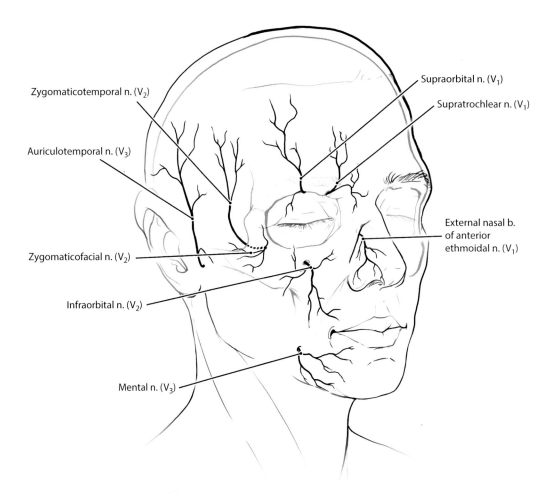

FIGURE 7.6   Branches of the trigeminal nerve (cranial nerve V).

rami that arborize, and therefore when these nerves are cut permanent deficits are rare or temporary.

iv. Marginal mandibular branch innervates orbicularis oris, depressor anguli oris, depressor labii inferioris, mentalis, and platysma muscles.

v. Cervical branch innervates the platysma muscle.

G. Danger zones for facial nerve injury

1. Temporal nerve branch of the facial nerve innervates the forehead.

Transection of the temporal branch of the facial nerve results in frontalis muscle paralysis.

a. Temporal nerve is most susceptible to injury within a triangle where upper border extends from the tragus to 2 cm above the lateral eyebrow and where lower border extends from the tragus across the superior malar eminence to the orbital rim (Figure 7.7).

b. Temporal nerve courses just beneath the superficial musculoaponeurotic system (SMAS).

c. Injury to the temporal branch results in forehead paralysis with a lack of wrinkling and eyebrow ptosis.

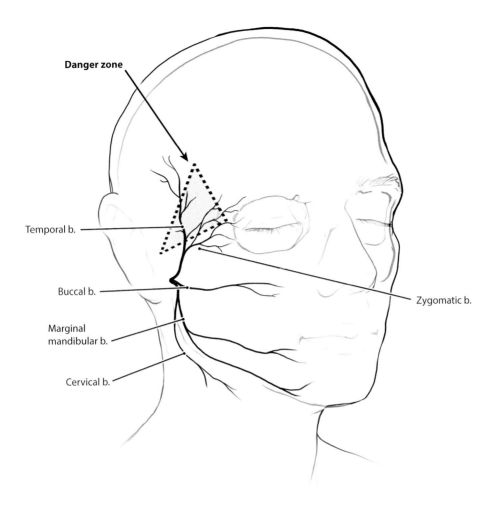

Danger zone

Temporal b.

Buccal b.

Marginal
mandibular b.

Cervical b.

Zygomatic b.

FIGURE 7.7 Branches of the facial nerve (cranial nerve VII). Note the triangular area where the temporal branches of the facial nerve are easily injured because of their superficial location. Injury to these nerves results in brow paralysis.

2. Marginal mandibular nerve branch of facial nerve innervates lower lip (Figure 7.8).
   a. Note that the marginal mandibular nerve crosses over the facial artery where the facial artery courses superiorly as it wraps around the mandible over a slight bone depression called the antegonial notch.
   b. Marginal mandibular nerve becomes superficial and most susceptible to injury 2 cm posterior to oral commissure. However, there is a great anatomic variability in exact position of this nerve.
   c. Injury results in paralysis of lower lip with drooling and an asymmetric smile. Patients cannot pull the damaged lip down or evert vermillion on the side of the nerve damaged.
3. Erb's point is located in the posterior triangle where the cervical plexus emerges deep to the midpoint of the posterior border of the sternocleidomastoid muscle. The cervical plexus contains the lesser occipital, great auricular, transverse cervical, and supraclavicular nerves.[4]
   a. The great auricular nerve (C_2, C_3) exits superficial to the cervical plexus from about the posterior midpoint of the sternocleidomastoid muscle and courses across the muscle anteriorly and superiorly to innervate most of the ear. Injury to this nerve results in ear numbness.

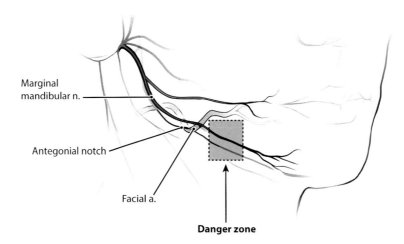

FIGURE 7.8 Course of marginal mandibular nerve which superficially crosses the facial artery near the margin of the mandible. Note the danger zone where the nerve is superficial and can be damaged. Damage to this nerve results in a crooked smile from muscle paralysis to the lateral lower lip.

      b. Spinal accessory nerve (XI), which innervates the trapezius muscle is at high risk of injury in this area. It exits from the posterior border of the sternocleidomastoid muscle above the point of exit of the great auricular nerve. It then courses posteriorly and inferiorly in the posterior cervical triangle to innervate the trapezius muscle. Damage to this nerve results in a winged scapula, arm paresthesias, impaired arm abduction, and a "frozen" shoulder.

  H. Facial nerve blocks

    1. Supraorbital nerve block anesthetizes the forehead and frontal scalp.

      a. The foramen from which this nerve emerges can be palpated along the superior orbital rim at the midpupillary line. The midpupillary line is an imaginary vertical line extending inferiorly from the center of the pupil with the patient gazing up so as to fix the pupil in the middle of the open eye.

    2. Infraorbital nerve block anesthetizes the medial cheek, upper lip, nasal ala, and lower eyelid.

      a. The foramen from which this nerve emerges is located about 1 cm below the inferior orbital rim on the midpupillary line. The infraorbital nerve can also be anesthetized intraorally between the upper first and second premolars in the midpupillary line.

    3. Mental nerve block anesthetizes the lower lip and part of the chin.

      a. The foramen from which this nerve emerges is on the mandible inferior to the lower second premolar.

      b. The foramen is located on the midpupillary line. Infraoral anesthetic administration is between the lower first and second premolars.

  I. Vascular supply of the face (Figure 7.9)

    1. Arterial supply to facial skin is supplied from a subdermal plexus that originates from branches of the internal and external carotid arteries. In general, the upper central face is supplied by branches of the internal carotid artery, whereas the lateral and lower faces are supplied by branches of the external carotid artery.

      a. The ophthalmic artery branch of the internal carotid artery sub-divides into the supraorbital, supratrochlear, dorsal nasal, and anterior ethmoidal artery to supply the upper central face.

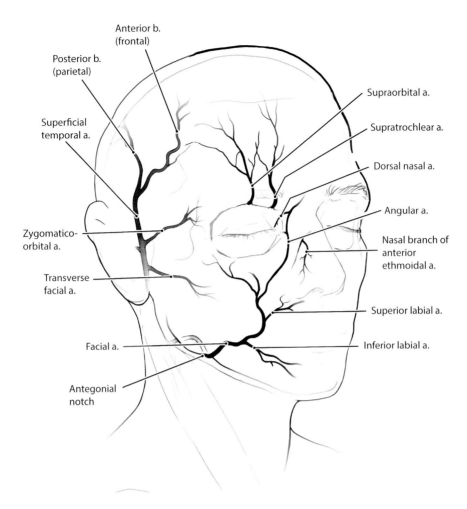

FIGURE 7.9 Main superficial arteries to the face.

b. Near the medial canthus, the dorsal nasal artery anastomoses with the angular artery which in turn comes off the facial artery.

c. The facial artery supplies a large portion of the anterior face. After branching from the external carotid artery, it courses through the submandibular salivary gland and below the mandible. The facial artery emerges over the midportion of the mandible (over the antegonial notch) coursing anteriorly and superiorly (Figure 7.8).

d. The inferior labial artery branches from the facial artery and courses below the lip while the superior labial artery branches from the facial artery above the lip. The facial artery continues superiorly onto the nose where it is known as the angular artery.

e. The angular artery anastomoses with the dorsal nasal artery just above the medial canthal tendon in the medial canthus.[5] Since the angular artery is a terminal branch from the external carotid artery and the dorsal nasal artery is a branch from the internal carotid artery, this anastomosis connects the internal and external carotid artery systems.

The anastomosis in the medial canthus of the angular artery and the dorsal nasal artery connects the internal to the external carotid artery systems.

f. The external carotid artery, after giving off the facial artery, courses superiorly below the ear where it gives off the posterior auricular artery. Anterior to the ear the external carotid artery becomes the superficial temporal artery. Here it gives off the transverse facial artery and zygomatico-orbital artery to supply the lateral face. The superficial temporal artery then continues superiorly and divides in the temporal scalp into an anterior (frontal) branch that supplies the forehead and a posterior (parietal) branch that supplies the lateral scalp.

2. Facial veins.

a. Facial veins, unlike veins elsewhere, lack valves and permit backflow of venous blood.

b. The facial vein connects to the deep facial vein at the cheek. The facial vein parallels the course of the facial artery.

c. The deep facial vein drains into the internal jugular vein which connects with the external jugular vein.

d. The deep facial vein communicates with the cavernous sinus of the brain through the pterygoid plexus. The pterygoid plexus drains the paranasal face and upper cutaneous lip. Skin or wound infections of the central face can gain access to the cavernous sinus through the pterygoid plexus.

e. The ophthalmic vein drains directly into the cavernous sinus.

f. The infraorbital vein drains into the cavernous sinus either through the pterygoid plexus or via the ophthalmic vein to which it connects.[3]

II. Hand

A. Innervation

1. Median nerve – located in the medial ventral wrist.

a. Sensory innervation of most of the palm and the palmar side and nailbeds of the thumb, index, and middle finger. The median nerve innervates half of the radial side of the palmar ring finger.

b. Motor innervation of the muscles are involved in fine precision functions of the hand.

c. Nerve block can be done but is difficult as nerve lies deep beneath fascia between palmaris longus and flexor carpi ulnaris tendons. Locate these tendons in the wrist by flexing the wrist. Inject 1 cm proximal to the wrist crease at a 45-degree angle ulnaris to palmaris.

2. Ulnar nerve – located in the lateral (ulnar) third of the ventral wrist

a. Sensory innervation of the palmar and dorsal sides of the fifth digit and the medial half of the ring finger.

b. Motor innervation to the muscles involved in grasping function of the hand.

c. Nerve lies deep to flexor carpi ulnaris and just lateral to the ulnar artery. Difficult to anesthetize. Risk of injury to nerve.

3. Radial nerve – located in the mid dorsal wrist, slightly radially

a. Sensory innervation of the radial aspect of the dorsum of the hand, thumb, and index finger. Sensory innervation of the third digit and the radial half of the ring finger proximal to the distal interphalangeal joints.

b. Motor innervation of the wrist extensors that control hand position and stabilization.

c. Generally not necessary to block as skin is loose on dorsum of hand.

B. Radial and ulnar arteries provide blood supply for the hand through forming superficial and deep palmar arches.

1. Dorsal and ventral neurovascular bundles course along the lateral sides of the fingers forming multiple anastomoses.

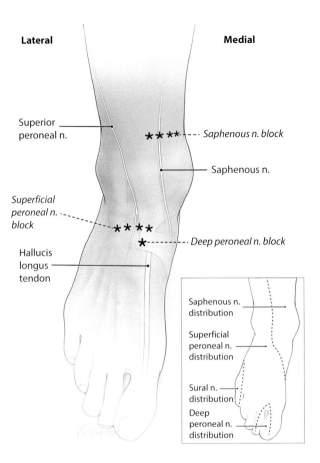

FIGURE 7.10 Anterior ankle for nerve block anesthesia. Suggested locations for nerve blocks indicated by *'s. Nerve distributions of dorsal foot shown on inset.

III. Foot
    A. Innervation
        1. Dorsum of foot (Figure 7.10).
            a. Superficial peroneal nerve – extends superficially over the dorsum of the foot.
                i. Innervates skin on dorsal foot.
                ii. Inject superficially across the dorsum of foot just distal to the ankle.
                iii. Because the skin on the dorsal foot is relatively loose, it is usually unnecessary to block this nerve.
            b. Deep peroneal nerve – lies medially at the bifurcation of the tibialis anterior tendon and the extensor hallucis longus tendon, the tendon to the great toe.
                i. Innervates skin between the first and second toes.
                ii. Nerve block is performed as shown in Figure 7.10. Inject deeply just lateral to extensor hallucis longus tendon.
            c. Saphenous nerve.
                i. Innervates medial posterior ventral foot and arch.
                ii. Nerve block performed as shown in Figure 7.10 by injections just above the medial malleolis in a horizontal direction medially.

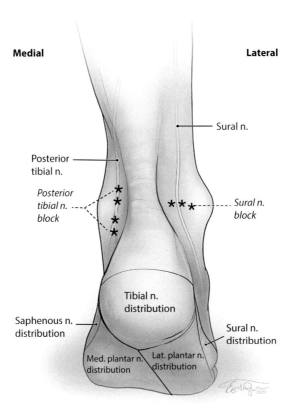

FIGURE 7.11   Posterior ankle for nerve block anesthesia. Suggested locations for nerve blocks indicated by *'s. Nerve distributions indicated on bottom of foot.

2. Ventral foot (sole).
    a. Posterior tibial nerve (Figure 7.11).
        i.   Branches into medial calcanean, medial plantar, and lateral plantar nerves. Innervates most of the ventral foot and heel.
        ii. Lies posterior to the medial malleolus, slightly posterior and lateral to posterior tibial artery.
        iii. Inject superiorly and inferiorly along this nerve so that the anesthesia will include the inferior branches (medial calcanean, medial and lateral plantar nerves).
    b. Sural nerve.
        i.   Innervates the lateral heel and posterior lateral ventral foot and dorsal lateral foot.
        ii. Situated on lateral posterior lower leg, runs inferiorly between Achilles tendon and lateral malleolus. Then, it descends below the lateral malleolus and courses anteriorly along the lateral foot and little toe.
        iii. Inject between Achilles tendon and lateral malleolus.

Conclusion

Anatomy is the cornerstone of dermatologic surgery. Surgical planning with respect to anatomical structures and landmarks is essential. Surface anatomy guides the dermatologist to avoid neural and vascular structures deep to anatomic landmarks. Judicious surgical design and execution facilitates optimal surgical results.

REFERENCES

1. Leffell DJ, Brown M. Manual of Skin Surgery: A Practical Guide to Dermatologic Procedures. 2nd Edition. People's Medical Publishing House, CT, 2011.
2. Mariwalla K, Leffell DJ. Primer in Dermatologic Surgery: A Study Companion. American Society for Dermatologic Surgery, IL, 2009.
3. Hollinshead W. Anatomy for Surgeons, Volume 1. Harper & Row Publishers, Philadelphia, PA, 1982; p. 145, 303.
4. Landers JT, Maino K. Clarifying Erb's Point as an Anatomic Landmark in the Posterior Cervical Triangle. Dermatol Surg 2012; 38(6): 954–957.
5. Williams P, Warwick R. Gray's Anatomy. 36th Edition. W. B. Saunders Company, Philadelphia, PA, 1980; p. 679.

8

Electrosurgery

Austin Liu and Naomi Lawrence

Introduction

Electrosurgery refers to the use of electricity to heat tissue during surgery. There are two forms of electrosurgery: (1) high-frequency electrosurgery (HFE) and (2) electrocautery. HFE is a modality that passes a controlled high-frequency alternating electric current through tissue. Tissue heat is generated by tissue resistance to electric current flow and results in heat damage. The other form of electrosurgery is electrocautery, which is used infrequently. In electrocautery, an electrical current passes through the electrode tip that becomes red hot by its resistance to current flow. When applied to tissue, the hot electrode tip directly transfers heat and thus causes heat damage. Unlike HFE, electrocautery does not pass an electrical current into tissue.[1]

In addition to providing hemostasis, both HFE and electrocautery can be used to "burn off" benign and malignant skin lesions and to debulk large tissues growths. The different forms of HFE include electrodesiccation, electrofulguration, electrocoagulation, and electrosection.[1] Each type of HFE has a typical current waveform, current strength, and voltage strength that results in a unique depth and breadth of tissue destruction (Table 8.1).

The machines available to generate HFE current are varied but usually capable of producing most or all forms of HFE. The development of HFE machines during the early 1900s by W.T. Bovie was a major advance in surgery, providing surgeons with an efficient and controlled method to stop bleeding by heating tissue.[2] The name "Bovie" is often used as a verb, as in "to bovie", meaning to apply an HFE current into tissue to stop bleeding or as an adjective applied to the electrosurgical machines which are then loosely known as "bovie machines". One brand of inexpensive electrosurgical machines commonly used by dermatologists is the Hyfrecator® (**HI**gh **FRE**quency eradi**CATOR**). This machine is a low-power electrosurgical machine that uses electrodesiccation and electrofulguration to remove superficial skin lesions such as warts, seborrheic keratosis etc.

> The verb "to bovie" in surgery has come to mean to apply HFE current to tissue to stop bleeding.

I. Pre-operative Evaluation

    A. Review medical history to assess risks associated with electric current flow in tissue.

        1. Pacemakers, cardiac defibrillators, deep-brain stimulators, and other implantable electronic devices (IED) (if not shielded properly) can malfunction, be activated, or reset with the use of HFE. A pacemaker can be temporarily disabled with an overlying magnet but the patient needs to have a cardiac monitor while the pacemaker is disabled.

           a. For an implanted pacemaker without a defibrillator the following are recommended.

              i. Use short bursts.

              ii. Avoid using electrode near pacemaker.

              iii. Place indifferent electrode so current will not flow through pacemaker.

> Be warned: it is possible to activate an implanted cardiac pacemaker/defibrillator with HFE current.

TABLE 8.1

High-Frequency Electrosurgery Forms

	Electrocutting	**Electrocoagulation**	**Electrofulguration**	**Electrodesiccation**
Waveform	Sinusoidal	Nonsinusoidal	Nonsinusoidal	Nonsinusoidal
Current Flow	High	Very high	Very low	Low
Voltage	Low	Very low	Very high	High
Tissue Destruction	Superficial	Deep	Superficial	Superficial
Monoterminal (M)/ Biterminal(B)	B	B	M	M

    b. For pacemaker with defibrillator, the following choices are recommended.

        i. Use electrocautery (pure heated electrode only, no tissue electricity).

        ii. Use "bipolar" forceps (electric current transmitted mainly between two tissue-contacting tips).

        iii. Temporarily disable pacemaker/defibrillator with an overlying magnet and monitor patient's heart rate while HFE is being used.

  B. Assess risk for excessive bleeding

    1. A patient on an anticoagulant or with a bleeding diathesis history may require more extensive and thorough electrosurgical hemostasis.

II. Monoterminal and Biterminal HFE

  A. Monoterminal

    1. A small active electrode tip is used to concentrate current and deliver it into tissue. There is no indifferent electrode (Figure 8.1A). Note that in all forms of electrosurgery (both HFE and electrocautery) the size of the electrode tip in contact with

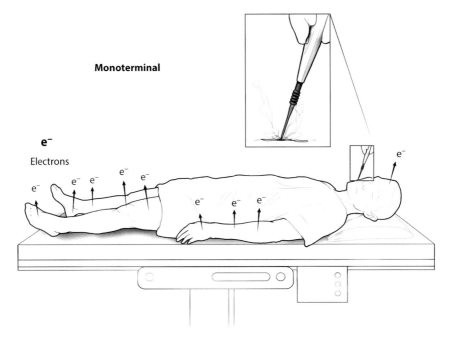

Monoterminal

FIGURE 8.1A Monoterminal high-frequency electrosurgery. Note small active electrode tip and no large second indifferent electrode plate. Electrons shed from patient to surrounding atmosphere.

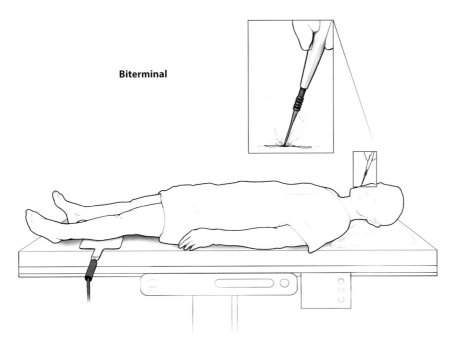

Biterminal

FIGURE 8.1B Biterminal high-frequency electrosurgery. Note small active electrode tip and large second indifferent (or dispersive) electrode plate under leg.

     the tissue determines the energy density and thus the subsequent degree of tissue destruction. At a given output setting, a fine electrode tip will produce concentrated tissue destruction whereas a broad electrode tip will produce less concentrated tissue destruction.[3]

  2. Monoterminal HFE types include electrodesiccation and electrofulguration.

  3. Monoterminal HFE is a less efficient method to heat tissue compared to biterminal HFE because current flow in tissue is low. In addition, the voltage is high and the current is markedly damped (nonsinusoidal).

  4. Electrode tip is not heated.

B. Biterminal

  1. Uses two electrodes: one with a small tip (the active electrode) that concentrates the current when touching the tissue and a second (indifferent or dispersive) electrode with a large surface area that diffuses the current. This second electrode is applied to the skin at a distant site and completes the electrical circuit back to the HFE machine (Figure 8.1B). The second electrode is large, usually a metal plate or a sticky gel pad, and must be in contact with a large portion of skin.

  2. Biterminal HFE types include electrocoagulation and electrosection.

  3. Biterminal HFE is a more efficient method to heat tissue compared to monoterminal HFE because tissue current flow is stepped-up by means of the second dispersive electrode that captures the current and its cord returns the current to the HFE machine to complete the circuit. This stepped-up current flow requires a lower voltage than that required for monotermined electrosurgery and uses a moderately damped current (electrocoagulation) or an undamped (sinusoidal) current (electrosection).

  4. Electrode tip is not heated.

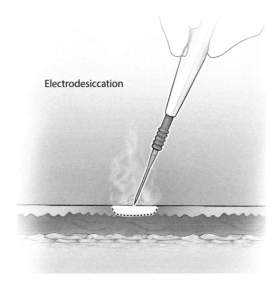

Electrodesiccation

FIGURE 8.2A Electrodesiccation. Note fine sparks and superficial tissue destruction.

III. Types of HFE (see Table 8.1)

    A. Electrodesiccation (see Figure 8.2A)

        1. Main characteristic – Superficial (epidermal) tissue destruction due to dehydration and vaporization.

           a. Minimal risk of scarring.

           b. Active electrode contacts the skin and may emit small fine sparks.

        2. Monoterminal device with damped low current flow and high voltage.

        3. Indications.

           a. Hemostasis – works best when applied to absolutely dry tissue field.

           b. To burn off superficial benign lesions such as seborrheic keratoses, dermatosis papulosa nigrans, warts, etc.

           c. Used after curettage to destroy remaining roots of superficial malignant growths, such as small squamous cell carcinomas in situ and small superficial basal cell carcinomas.

> Electrodesiccation is one of the most frequently misspelled words in medicine. Remember it has two "Cs" and one "S" from the Latin word *sicca* meaning dry. Compare with sicca syndrome.

    B. Electrofulguration (see Figure 8.2B)

        1. Main characteristic – superficial tissue destruction via sparks. The sparks heat tissue and cause dehydration and carbonization; the latter appears as tissue char.

           a. Active electrode tip does not need to come into contact with tissue.

               i. Active electrode tip is kept 1–2 millimeters away from the tissue.

           b. Sparks arc from electrode directly onto tissue.

           c. Sparks are less controllable and larger than those with electrodesiccation. Thus, tissue destruction is slightly wider and slightly deeper than that with electrodesiccation.

        2. Monoterminal device with damped slightly higher current flow and higher voltage than that with electrodesiccation.

        3. Indications same as for electrodesiccation.

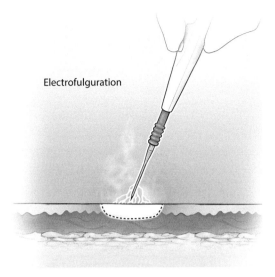

FIGURE 8.2B   Electrofulguration. Note tip does not need to touch tissue and sparks are large and not easily controlled. Tissue destruction is slightly wider and deeper than that with electrodesiccation.

C. Electrocoagulation (see Figure 8.2C)

  1. Main characteristic – Deeper tissue destruction than that resulting from electrodesiccation or electrofulguration (see Figure 8.2C).

    a. Tissue charring should be minimized to decrease scarring and risk of infection.

    b. Can grasp tissue with metal forceps and touch the active electrode tip to forceps. The current flows down the metal forceps and coagulates tissue between the tips of the forceps. Note that with electrodesiccation or electrofulguration, because of low current flow, current will not flow down metal forceps that grasp tissue.

    c. Very small sparks can occur.

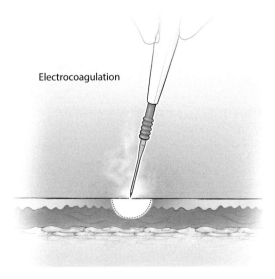

FIGURE 8.2C   Electrocoagulation. Note the deeper tissue destruction than that with electrodesiccation or electrofulguration.

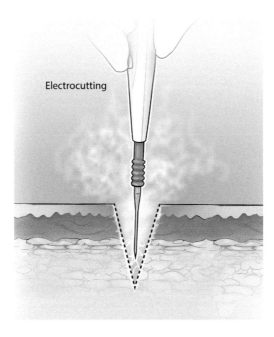

FIGURE 8.2D Electrocutting (electrotomy, electrosection). Note the large smoke plume.

2. Biterminal device with moderately damped high current flow that requires a low voltage. Thus, electrocoagulation uses a large indifferent second electrode in addition to the small active electrode tip.

3. Indications: same as for electrodesiccation and electrofulguration. However, for hemostasis, electrocoagulation is more efficient and more powerful than electrodesiccation or electrofulguration.

D. Electrocutting (electrotomy, electrosection) (see Figure 8.2D)

1. Main characteristic – vaporizes tissue with minimal surrounding heat damage.

a. Can cut tissue and seal surrounding blood vessels simultaneously.

b. Prominent smoke plume with tissue vaporization.

2. Biterminal device with undamped (sinusoidal) high current flow requiring a low voltage.

3. Indications.

a. Cutting through skin.

b. Excision of pendulous or sessile skin growths, e.g., neurofibromas, verrucae etc.

c. Undermining skin.

d. Vascular lesion excision.

e. Rhinophyma paring and excision of acne keloidalis nuchae.

IV. Electrocautery

A. Definition: direct transference of heat to tissue; no electric current is transferred into the tissue.

B. Electric current is used to heat electrode tip, which causes coagulation/necrosis when it touches tissue. Thus, the electrode tip is red hot unlike HFE where the electrode tip is not heated. The operative field does not need to be completely dry to provide hemostasis by the hot electrode tip.

> In electrocautery the active electrode tip is heated, whereas in HFE the active electrode tip is not heated.

C. Indications
   1. Useful to provide hemostasis and to burn off small benign or superficial malignant lesions.
   2. Very useful when HFE is contraindicated as in a patient with an implantable electronic device (IED).
      a. Cardiac defibrillator.
      b. Implantable cardioverter defibrillator (ICD).
      c. Gastric pacemaker.
      d. Cochlear implant.
      e. Deep brains, nerve, spinal cord, bone stimulator.

V. Complications
   A. Scarring
      1. More likely with HFE current causing deep tissue destruction such as electrocoagulation.
   B. Malfunction of pacemaker/cardiac defibrillator/brain stimulator/other implantable electrical devices (IED).
      1. May occur with HFE. Interference and oversensing is more likely in the monoterminal mode than in the biterminal mode.[4]
      2. Electrocautery or "bipolar" forceps can be utilized to avoid interference with an IED.
      3. Modern cardiac pacemakers have more protection than older pacemakers from environmental electromagnetic inference (EMI). This protection includes improved electric shielding and filtering systems.
   C. Electrical shocks from electron shedding will occur with monoterminal electrosurgery if one touches the patient without rubber gloves during electrodesiccation or electrofulguration. Electric shocks to the patient can occur with biterminal HFE if patient is touching a small portion of the large indifferent electrode because the current intensifies as it localizes to a small skin area, or if the patient inadvertently touches metal attached to the operating table.
   D. Skin burns or fires are possible if sparks from the HFE electrode tip ignite alcohol-containing substances that have not dried after being applied preoperatively to the skin for disinfection (such as isopropyl alcohol, Hibiclens® [4% chlorhexidine gluconate with 4% isopropyl alcohol], or ChloraPrep [2% chlorhexidine gluconate with 70% isopropyl alcohol]).

   It is possible to cause a fire if sparks from the HFE electrode tip come in contact with a wet alcohol-containing disinfectant on the skin surface.

   E. Explosions or fires are possible if oxygen (which is flammable) is flowing during surgery. When HFE is used, oxygen should be turned off.
   F. Infection – surgical tips should be sterile. However, infection is unlikely as HFE surgical current acts as a sterilizing agent for bacteria.[5] The sterilizing effects of HFE on viruses (hepatitis, warts, HIV, or prion disease) is unknown. However, HPV (human papilloma virus) has been detected in the inevitable smoke plume produced by HFE.

Conclusion

Electrosurgery is important to provide hemostasis and as a destructive treatment modality for both benign and malignant lesions. Several forms of electrosurgery are available for the dermatologic surgeon. By taking into account the unique properties of each type of electrosurgery as well as the patient's medical risk factors, the surgeon can select the most appropriate device and current type to use.

REFERENCES

1. Soon SL, Washington CV. Electrosurgery, electrocoagulation, electrofulguration, electrodessication, electrosection, electrocautery. In: Surgery of the Skin: Procedural Dermatology (Robinson JK et al., editors). Elsevier, New York, 2010; 137–152.
2. Cushing H. Electro-surgery as an Aid to the Removal of Intracranial Tumors With a Preliminary Note on a New Surgical-Current Generator by W. T. Bovie. Surg Gynecol Obstet 1928; 47: 751–755.
3. Sebben JE. Cutaneous Electrosurgery. Year Book Medical Publishers, Chicago, 1989.
4. Taheri A, Mansoori P, Sandoval L et al. Electrosurgery: Part II. Technology, Applications, and Safety of Electrosurgical Devices. J Am Acad Dermatol 2014; 70: 607.e1–607.e12.
5. Bennett RG, Kraffert C. Bacterial Transference During Electrodessication and Electrocoagulation. Arch Derm 1990; 126: 751–755.

ABBREVIATIONS

HFE   High-frequency electrosurgery
IED   Implantable electronic device
ICD   Implantable cardioverter defibrillator

9

Dressings and Their Effects on Wound Healing

Ronald G. Wheeland

Introduction

Over the past several decades, basic research has provided important information about the processes involved in wound healing. No longer is dry wound healing acceptable because it results in wound bed desiccation, which increases the wound depth and wound healing time. To preclude these events, occlusive dressings have become standard. An occlusive dressing not only protects the wound from outside trauma and prevents wound desiccation but also continuously keeps the locally produced growth factors in contact with the wound base to maximize their stimulatory effects on keratinocytes, fibroblasts, and blood vessels. An occlusive dressing minimizes the amount of wound care often required and reduces discomfort. The many benefits of occlusive wound dressings have led to the development of several new surgical dressings that speed wound healing and improve the final scar appearance.

I. Concept of Keeping Wound Moist
   A. A moist wound heals faster and with less scar than a dry wound.[1,2]
   B. If a crust or scab develops on a wound, the regenerating epidermis has to navigate a path underneath the crust which takes longer and results in a deeper wound due to loss of superficial dermis (Figure 9.1).
II. Traditional Dressing (Figure 9.2)
   A. Covers the wound, absorbs wound drainage, provides compression, and maintains moist environment. Plays no active role in wound healing and epidermal regeneration.
   B. Anatomy of a traditional dressing. Its component parts include:
      1. Contact layer. Usually an ointment which provides lubrication to minimize wound disruption and desiccation and to allow the overlying dressing to be easily removed, e.g., sterile petroleum jelly (Vaseline®), or sterile antibiotic ointment (e.g., Polysporin®) (Table 9.1). Another alternative contact layer is gauze impregnated with petroleum jelly (Vaseline™ gauze [Covidien]) or gauze impregnated with an antibacterial agent such as 3% bismuth tribromophenate (Xeroform® [Covidien]). Another gauze-like contact layer commonly used is Adaptic™ (Acelity), which is made with cellulose acetate and a petroleum emulsion. Vaseline® gauze is hydrophobic whereas Adaptic™ or Xeroform® gauze is hydrophilic.
      2. Absorbent non-stick pad. Placed on top of the ointment. Non-stick gauze reduces trauma to epidermal cells at the wound base during dressing changes. Usually the "non-stick" bandage has absorbent cellulose between two layers of perforated polyester film with small holes (e.g., Telfa™ [Covidien]). The cellulose wicks drainage from the wound through holes in the polyester film.

(a)

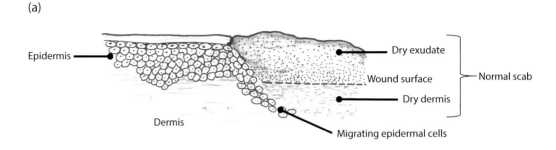

(b)

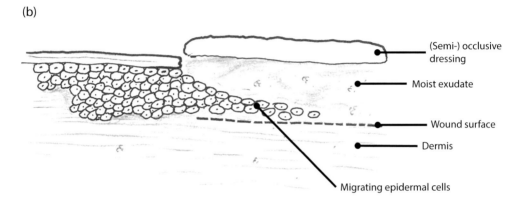

FIGURE 9.1 Epidermal cells migrating to cross wound. If scab is present (A) epidermal cells must go deeper to avoid scab formation than if wound is kept moist (B). (Reproduced with permission from Bennett RG, *Fundamentals of Cutaneous Surgery*, C.V. Mosby, St. Louis, 1988.)

    3. Cushioning layer. Usually gauze applied directly or unfolded and fluffed. Helps to add bulk and put pressure on a wound.

    4. Tape. Flesh tone paper type is preferred as it is nonallergenic and the color helps to camouflage the dressing. Cut tape looks neat and gives the message that the underlying surgery was done with meticulous care. Tape is generally placed in the direction of the maximum skin tension lines.

> Always cut the tape on a dressing rather than tearing it; cut tape looks neater than torn tape.

  III. Synthetic Dressing Materials – useful when traditional wound dressings fail to heal a wound (Table 9.2).

    A. Polyurethane membranes – composed of a self-adhesive polyurethane sheet permeable to oxygen, CO_2, and water vapor moisture from the wound, but is impermeable to water, wound exudate, or bacteria.

      1. Physical appearance: transparent or semitransparent thin sheet.

      2. Various products: Opsite (Smith & Nephew), Tegaderm (3M), Tegaderm Film (3M), Bioclusive (Johnson & Johnson), Acu-Derm (Acme United), UniFlex (Smith & Nephew), Blisterfilm (Covidien), Polyskin (Covidien), and Visulin (Hartmann).

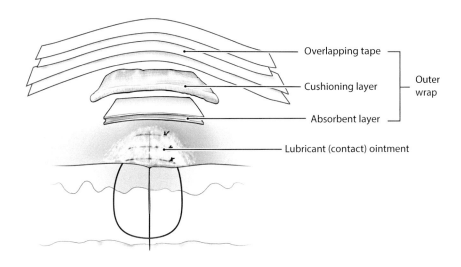

FIGURE 9.2 Anatomy of a traditional dressing. The contact layer can be either ointment alone or gauze with ointment. (Reproduced with permission from Bennett RG, *Fundamentals of Cutaneous Surgery*, C.V. Mosby, St. Louis, 1988.)

TABLE 9.1

Topical Wound Ointments and Creams with and without Antibiotics

Product	Ingredient	Antimicrobial Spectrum
Vaseline[®b]	White petrolatum	None
Aquaphor[®c]	41% petrolatum, mineral oil, lanolin	None
Bacitracin ointment	Bacitracin	*Streptococcus, Staphylococcus*
Neosporin® ointment	Neomycin sulfate, polymyxin B, bacitracin	Proteus, *E. coli,* gram-negative rods
Polysporin® ointment	Polymyxin B sulfate/ bacitracin	Pseudomonas, *E. coli*, gram-negative rods except Proteus
Bactroban® ointment or Centany® ointment	Mupirocin calcium	MRSA[a], other *Staphylococcus, Streptococcus*, some gram negatives
Gentamycin ointment[d]	Gentamycin sulfate	*Staphylococcus, E. coli*, Proteus, Pseudomonas
Fucidin® ointment	Sodium fusidate	*Staphylococcus*
Silver sulfadiazine (Silvadene®) cream	Silver sulfadiazine	Pseudomonas, Enterobacter, *Staphylococcus*, Beta-Hemolytic Streptococcus
Mafenide (Sulfamylon®) cream	Mafenide acetate	Pseudomonas, some anaerobic bacteria

[a] Methicillin-resistant *Staphylococcus aureus*.
[b] Available in sterile and nonsterile forms.
[c] Available only in nonsterile form.
[d] Cross reacts with neomycin.

3. Prevent desiccation of wound base.
4. Keep wounds hydrated.
5. Retain growth factors at wound site.

TABLE 9.2

Synthetic Wound Dressings

Dressing Type	Adherent	Absorbent	Actions	Examples
Polyurethane Sheet	Yes	No	Creates moist environment	Opsite, Tegaderm
Hydrocolloid	Yes	Yes	Absorbs wound drainage, autolytic debridement	Duoderm
Hydrogel	No	No	Cooling effect, adds moisture	Vigilon
Polyurethane Foam	No	Yes	Absorbs drainage	Mepilex
Plastic Mesh	No	No	Maintains moisture	N-Terface
Silicone with Nylon in Gel	No	No	Minimizes elevated scars	Mepitel, Cica-care
Cellulose between polyester film layers	No	Yes	Maintains moisture	Telfa

     6. Stimulate cellular effects locally.

     7. Do not absorb wound drainage. Thus, fluid can accumulate underneath the dressing and leak at the dressing edges.

     8. Indications: laceration, abrasions, split thickness skin graft donor site wounds, to hold pinch grafts in place,[3] Mohs surgery wounds.[4]

     9. Contraindications: wounds with heavy exudate, infected wounds.

  B. Hydrocolloid dressings – composed of methylcellulose, gelatin, or pectin which are hydrophilic and impermeable to oxygen and water.

     1. Physical appearance: opaque sheet.

     2. Various products: DuoDERM® (ConvaTec) DuoDERM®CGF™ (ConvaTec), DuoDERM® Extra Thin (ConvaTec), Comfeel® (Coloplast), 3M Tegasorb™ (AliMed), Restore (Hollister), Intrasite (Smith & Nephew), Ultec™ (Kendall).

     3. Provide excellent autolytic debridement of necrotic tissue in the wound base.

     4. Reduce the amount of tissue necrosis and depth of scar.

     5. Speed re-epidermization and re-epithelialization.

     6. Absorb wound secretions which results in gel formation.

     7. Can be left in place for several days.

     8. Indications: chronic wounds, wounds where dressing change is hard to do daily. Good physical barrier that provide wound protection from outside bacteria.

  C. Hydrogel dressings – composed of methacrylates, polyvinylpyrrolidone, gelatin, pectin, chitosan.

     1. Physical appearance: semitransparent gel.

     2. Various products: Vigilon (Bard), Cutinova (Smith & Nephew), Elasto-Gel (SouthWest), Geliperm (Geistlich Sons Ltd), Nu-Gel (Systagenix), and Intrasite Gel (Smith & Nephew).

     3. Minimize trauma to new epidermal cells at wound base.

     4. Maintain wound hydration.

     5. Have a cooling effect and are thus soothing for superficial wounds following dermabrasion or laser abrasion.[5]

     6. Indications: post dermabrasion or laser abrasion. Also useful for large superficial abrasion ("brush burn" or "rug burn").

     7. Contraindications: heavy wound exudate, infected wounds.

  D. Polyurethane foams – composed of polyurethane sponge

     1. Physical appearance: sponge-like.

2. Various products: Lyofoam® Max (Mölnlyck®), Mepilex XT (Mölnlyck®).

3. Semipermeable: allow water vapor to enter but provide a barrier to bacteria.

4. Absorb wound drainage.

5. Indications: very exudative wound.

IV. Unique Dressings

   A. N-Terface® (Alimed)[6]

      1. High density mesh woven with monofilament polyethylene threads.

      2. Non-adherent, permeable material.

      3. Minimizes trauma and pain of dressing changes.

      4. Prevents mechanical disruption of re-epithelializing wounds.

      5. Indications: split-thickness skin graft donor wounds, open wounds.

   B. Silicone dressings

      1. Available products: silicone-coated nylon (Mepitel Nonadherent Silicone Dressing [Mölnlycke]), silicone gel sheeting (Cica-care [Smith & Nephew], Epi-Derm [Biodermis]).

      2. Nonadherent.

      3. Help shrink keloids and hypertrophic scars.

      4. Reduce pain and itching of keloids and hypertrophic scars.

> Silicone dressings may mysteriously lessen hypertrophic scars and keloids.

      5. Reduce erythema.

      6. Mechanism unknown.

         a. May trap growth factors like tumor necrosis factor (TNF) locally and reduce collagen.

         b. May increase local tissue temperature resulting in tissue injury or increased vascularity.

         c. May increase pressure and thus physically counteract excess scar formation.

         d. May help retain moisture on scar tissue.

         e. May reduce collagen formation.

      7. Indications: hypertrophic scars or keloids, pruritic scars.

   C. Alginate dressings [7,8]

      1. A "phytogenetic" dressing composed of nonwoven fibers of cellulose-like polysaccharide derived from brown seaweed. Contains sodium/calcium salts of alginic acid as well as zinc, magnesium.

      2. Available products: Calcium Alginate Dressings SHEET (McKesson), Kaltostat (ConvaTec), Algosteril (Smith & Nephew), Sorbsan (Pharma-Plast Ltd).

      3. May be combined with hydrocolloid (e.g., Comfeel Alginate Dressing [Coloplast]) or silver (e.g., Calcium Alginate Dressings SHEET with Ag [McKesson]).

      4. Non-adherent.

      5. Highly absorbent.

      6. Form hydrophilic gel when in contact with wound exudate. Exchange of calcium ions from dressing with sodium ions from wound results in gel formation.

      7. Stimulate autolytic debridement.

      8. Provide hemostasis for bleeding wounds.

      9. Indications: excessive wound drainage, hemostasis.

      10. Contraindications: dry wounds, deep sinuses.

D. Paraffin dressings
  1. Gauze impregnated with paraffin.
  2. Available products: Jelonet (Smith & Nephew).
  3. Non-stick gauze.
  4. Indications: contact layer on sutured wound or open wound.

E. Antimicrobial dressings
  1. Available products: silver (Calcium Alginate Dressings SHEET with Ag [McKesson], Mepilex Ag [Mölnlycke], Contreet [Coloplast Corp], Algidex™ Ag [AliMed]); iodine (Inadine [Systagenix]); cadexomer iodine (Iodoflex [Smith & Nephew]); povidine-iodine containing hydrogel (Repithel® [Mundipharma Medical Company]); petroleum gauze with 3% bismuth tribromophenate (Xeroform® [Covidien]).
  2. Minimize wound bacterial colonization.
  3. Indications: chronically infected wounds.

V. Biologic and Bioengineered Dressing Materials[9],[10]

A. Skin substitutes – sometimes used for temporary coverage until autografting is possible. Result in lesser tendency toward excessive granulation tissue formation and lead to softer scars.

B. "Bioengineered" dressings combine biologic tissues and man-made materials. These dressing materials are broadly grouped into two categories:
  1. Dermoinductive – provide living cells into the wound that stimulate new tissue growth and granulation (e.g., Apligraf®).
  2. Dermoconductive – provides a cellular collagen scaffolding allowing surrounding tissue cells to migrate into the dressing structure (e.g., Alloderm®).

  > "Bioengineered" dressings are the new frontier in wound dressing materials.

C. Types (Table 9.3)

TABLE 9.3

Biologic and Bioengineered Wound Dressings

Dressing Type	Product	Composition
Autograft	Epicel	Patient's cultured keratinocytes
Allograft	Epifix®	Human amnion/chorion
	Affinity®	Human amnion/chorion
	Grafix®	Human placenta
	TheraSkin®	Human cadaver skin (epidermis and dermis)
	Graft-Jacket™[b]	Human cadaver acellular dermal matrix
	Alloderm™[b]	Human cadaver acellular dermal matrix
Xenograft	EZ Derm®	Porcine dermis
	Oasis®[b]	Porcine small intestinal submucosa
	Matristem™[b]	Porcine urinary bladder
Allograft/xenograft	Apligraf®[a]	Bovine collagen + neonatal fibroblasts and keratinocytes
	OrCel®[a]	Bovine collagen + neonatal fibroblasts and keratinocytes
Synthetic/allograft	Transcyte™	Human fibroblasts + nylon mesh+ silastic layer (silicone + plastic)
	Dermagraft®[a]	Human fibroblasts + polyglactin 910
Synthetic/xenograft	Biobrane®[b]	Porcine collagen + silicone and nylon mesh
	Integra®[b]	Bovine collagen + shark glycosaminoglycan + silicone
Phytogenic	Talymed®	Fibers from microalgae
	Kaltostat®	Calcium or sodium alginate from brown seaweed

[a] Dermoinductive (contains living cells).[10]
[b] Dermoconductive (contains acellular collagen scaffold).[10]

1. Autograft.
    a. Cultured keratinocyte autografts.
        i. Composed of monolayer of autologous keratinocytes (patient's own cells) from small biopsy grown in cell culture. Culture takes 3 weeks.
        ii. Available products: Epicel (Vericel).
        iii. Cells are expanded into sheets and applied to large burn wounds or other open wounds.
        iv. Graft is delicate and susceptible to mechanical damage. Thus, not useful for pressure-bearing areas.
        v. Susceptible to infection.
        vi. Provides a functional, but not a cosmetically acceptable, result.
2. Allograft.
    a. Amniotic dressings.
        i. Constitutes innermost part of amniotic sac, composed of human amnion/chorion.
        ii. Available products: Epifix® (MiMedx Group Inc.), Affinity® (Organogenesis).
        iii. Thin and semipermeable tissue.
        iv. Obtained during a caesarean section.
        v. Composed of multiple layers of epithelial cells, a thick basement membrane, and avascular connective tissue matrix. The latter supplies extracellular matrix protein, growth factors, and cytokines to promote wound healing.
        vi. Relatively cheap.
    b. Placental membrane.
        i. Cellular matrix from human placental membrane.
        ii. Available product: Grafix (Osiris Therapeutics Inc.).
        iii. Has mesenchymal stem cells, neonatal fibroblasts, and epithelial cells.
        iv. Use: noninfected wounds.
    c. Human skin.
        i. Cryopreserved cadaver epidermis and dermis.
        ii. Available products: TheraSkin® (Lifenet Health).
        iii. Provides growth factors, cytokines, and collagen.
    d. Human collagen matrix.
        i. Human cadaver acellular dermal matrix.
        ii. Available products: Graft-Jacket™ (Wright Medical Group), Alloderm™ (LifeCell).
        iii. Dermal replacement.
3. Xenograft.
    a. Porcine dermis.
        i. Available products: EZ Derm® (Mölnlycke).
        ii. Protects against external bacterial infections and body fluid loss.
        iii. May transmit viruses such as porcine cytomegalovirus.
        iv. Always shed (rejected) prior to wound healing.
        v. Inexpensive.
        vi. Used as temporary dressing until reconstruction is done. Often used on burns where it is left for 3–4 days.

b.   Porcine small intestinal submucosa.
   i.   Available products: Oasis (Smith & Nephew).
   ii. Acellular matrix.
   iii. Acts as scaffold for cellular migration and vascularization.
   iv. Contraindicated in patients with porcine sensitivity.
c.   Porcine urinary bladder.
   i.   Intact basement membrane and collagen. Also contains glycosaminoglycans and growth factors.
   ii. Available product: Matristem™ (ACell Inc.).
   iii. Acellular matrix scaffold with acellular basement membrane.
   iv. Gradually resorbed.
   v.   For nonhealing wounds.
d.   Allograft/xenograft.
   i.   A bilayer composed of bovine type I collagen with human neonatal foreskin fibroblasts and human neonatal keratinocytes.
   ii. Available products: Apligraf® (Organogenesis) OrCel® (Medgadget).
   iii. Human keratinocytes cultured on human collagen.
   iv. Not for infected wounds.
   v.   Not for patients allergic to bovine collagen.
   vi. Very expensive.
   vii. Indications: large burns wounds, diabetic ulcers.
e.   Synthetic/allograft.
   i.   Cultured human neonatal fibroblasts on a synthetic substrate.
   ii. Available products: nylon mesh substrate with silicone/plastic layer (Transcyte™ [Organogenesis]), polyglactin 910 substrate (Dermagraft® [Organogenesis]).
f.   Synthetic/xenograft.
   i.   Porcine collagen.
      a) Available products: Biobrane (Smith & Nephew).
      b) A composite of different materials – silicone membrane and nylon mesh imbedded in porcine collagen.
      c) Helps retain wound moisture to decrease desiccation of wound base.
      d) Expensive.
   ii. Bovine collagen matrix.
      a) Available products: Integra® (Integra LifeSciences Corp.).
      b) A bilayer (bilaminar) dermal regenerative template composed of bovine collagen (with shark chondroiten-6-sulfate glycosaminoglycan) and silicone.
      c) Useful for covering avascular wounds such as bone cartilage and tendon for faster wound healing.
      d) Acts as a scaffold for fibroblastic and endothelial invasion.
      e) Bilayer structure provides for scaffold for infiltration of host cells to form neodermis in 3–6 weeks.
      f) At 3–6 weeks the silicone layer lifts off and a thin STSG can be applied. Produces sterile exudate normally.
      g) Steep learning curve.

        h) Not to be used in patients with allergy to bovine collagen.

        i)   Expensive.

        j)   Indications: temporary wound covering until reconstruction can be done. Useful as placeholder until margins checked pathologically.

   g. Phytogenic dressing.

      i.   Available products: Talymed® (Marine Polymer Technologies Inc.).

      ii. Composed of shortened fibers of poly-N-acetylglucosamine, isolated from microalgae, a photosynthetic eukaryotic organism.

VI. Clinical Uses of Surgical Dressings

  A. Polyurethane membranes

    1. Sutured wound at sites difficult to reach or see.

    2. Excellent for split-thickness skin graft donor sites.

    3. Hold and protect pinch grafts in chronic leg ulcer wounds.[3]

    4. Cover and protect ulcerative capillary hemangiomas.

    5. Excellent for superficial abrasions.

  B. Hydrocolloid dressings

    1. Debridement of decubitus ulcers.

    2. Debridement of chronic leg ulcers.

    3. Protection of sutured or open wounds from trauma.

    4. Speed re-epithelialization of ulcerative phase of infantile capillary hemangiomas.

  C. Silicone dressings

    1. Reduce size and symptoms of keloids.

    2. Reduce redness and elevation of hypertrophic scars.

    3. May trap "anti-growth" factors (TNF and FGF) at scar site.

  D. Biologic dressings

    1. Temporary dressing only.

    2. Prevent environmental bacterial colonization of wounds.

    3. Impede fluid loss.

    4. Useful for diabetic ulcers, burns, chronic lower extremity ulcers.

    5. Promised efficacy often does not match reality.

    6. Usually very expensive.

Conclusion

Occlusive or semi-occlusive dressings have demonstrated proven value in dermatologic surgery by reducing postoperative pain, speeding wound healing, and improving the final cosmetic result. In addition, their use for chronic wounds like decubitus ulcers and leg ulcers has reduced the cost over traditional dressings. By selecting the most ideal synthetic dressing or combination of synthetic dressings, caring for wounds of all types and causes has become easier and more effective.

REFERENCES

1. Fisher LB, Maibach HI. Physical Occlusion Controlling Epidermal Mitosis. J Invest Dermatol 1972; 59: 106–108.
2. Eaglstein WE, Davis SC, Mehle AL, Mertz PM. Optimal Use of an Occlusive Dressing to Enhance Healing. Arch Dermatol 1988; 124: 392–395.

3. Gilmore WA, Wheeland RG. Treatment of Ulcers on Legs by Pinch Grafts and a Support Dressing of Polyurethane. J Dermatol Surg Oncol 1982; 8: 177–183.

4. Hein NT, Prawer SE, Katz HI. Facilitated Wound Healing Using Transparent Film Dressing Following Mohs Micrographic Surgery. Arch Dermatol 1988; 124: 903–906.

5. Mandy SH. A New Primary Wound Dressing Made of Polyethylene Oxide Gel. J Dermatol Surg Oncol 1983; 9: 153–155.

6. Salasche SJ, Winton GB. Clinical Evaluation of a Nonadhering Wound Dressing. J Dermatol Surg Oncol 1986; 12: 1220–1222.

7. Gupta R, Foster ME, Miller E. Calcium Alginate in the Management of Acute Surgical Wounds and Abscesses. J Tissue Viability 1991; 1: 115–116.

8. Vermeulen H, Ubbink D, Goossens A et al. Dressings and Topical Agents for Surgical Wound Healing by Secondary Intention. Cochrane Database Syst Rev 2004; 2: CD003554.

9. Hughes OB, Rakosi A, Macquhae F et al. A Review of Cellular and Acellular Matrix Products: Indications, Techniques, and Outcomes. Plast Reconstr Surg 2016; 138: 138–147S.

10. Thorton JF, Carboy JA, editors. Cellular and Tissue-Based Wound Care in Facial Reconstruction after Mohs Surgery in Facial Reconstruction After Mohs Surgery. Thieme Publishers, New York, 2018; p. 22–27.

10

Basic Suturing and Excision Techniques

Kapila V. Paghdal and Murad Alam

Introduction

To produce the best possible scars with sutured wounds, physicians need to understand the fundamentals of excision and basic suturing. Also necessary for success is knowledge of the different suture materials and various stitch techniques.

I. Basic Excision Technique

    A. Excisions, in most cases, are planned in a fusiform shape where the direction of the long axis lies parallel to the maximum skin tension lines (Figures 10.1 and 10.2).

        1. The excision shape is marked on the skin with a gentian violet skin marker in the desired direction. It is also helpful for orientation to mark out nearby wrinkles and maximum skin tension lines.

        2. The reason for this shape and orientation is that the formation of standing cones (dog-ears) is minimized.

        3. The ideal length-to-width ratio is 3:1 with a 30-degree angle at each apex (Figure 10.3).

        4. Other excision shapes include:

            a. "S"-shaped (sometimes called "lazy S") excision (Figure 10.4 middle) which can be used on a convex area to prevent a tethered scar or on a concave area to prevent a tented scar.

            b. Crescentic-shaped excision (Figure 10.4 bottom) which can be used in areas such as the chin or malar eminence where a curved scar would parallel the crescentic maximum skin tension lines (see also Figure 10.1).

            c. An "M"-plasty can be used to shorten the length of the scar (Figure 10.5).

    B. The incision is usually done with a #15 blade on a No. 3 scalpel handle.

        1. Provide traction to stretch the skin with the thumb and index finger of the non-dominant hand.

        2. To cut the skin, use the belly of the blade at a 90-degree angle to the skin surface.

        3. Generally, the depth of incision is down to the subcutaneous fat but may extend deeper if necessary for complete excision.

        4. One end of the tissue to be excised is grasped with forceps so that the scalpel or scissors can cut the specimen base at an even depth until the tissue is freed from surrounding skin.

        5. Hemostasis is achieved with pressure, high-frequency electrosurgery, or ligation of any bleeding vessels.

        6. Undermining the wound edges separates lateral to the wound the dermis from underlying fat. This procedure lessens tension and allows precise epidermal/dermal

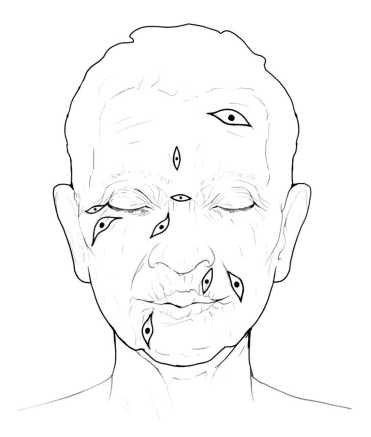

FIGURE 10.1 Fusiform excisions along facial maximum skin tension lines.

wound edge alignment when the two sides of the excision are brought together by sutures. Undermining is usually done with blunt tipped scissors, but sometimes a scalpel blade is necessary.

Remember that gentle tissue handling is an important principle when trying to produce the best possible scars.

   a. The wound edges are lifted with a skin hook or forceps. Be careful not to shred tissue with the skin hook or crush tissue with the forceps.

   b. Of note, planes of undermining are based on the area of the excision.

      i. In general, the level of undermining is the mid subcutaneous fat.

      ii. Scalp: subgaleal plane is preferred because it is relatively bloodless.

      iii. Lip/eyelid: above muscle.

   c. Before stitching, it is important to ensure that the wound edges are squared off at a 90-degree angle to the wound base and that bleeding is stopped.

      i. Ragged or inwardly slanted wound edges can result in imprecise epidermal/dermal apposition when sutured. Wound edge surfaces at different heights or apposition gaps in a sutured wound may result in an uneven or widened healed scar.

7. Depending on wound depth and wound edge tension, multiple layers of sutures may be necessary (i.e., fascial/deep buried, dermal/subcutaneous, epidermal/dermal). Generally, two layers of sutures are used: dermal/subcutaneous and epidermal/dermal.

(a) (b)

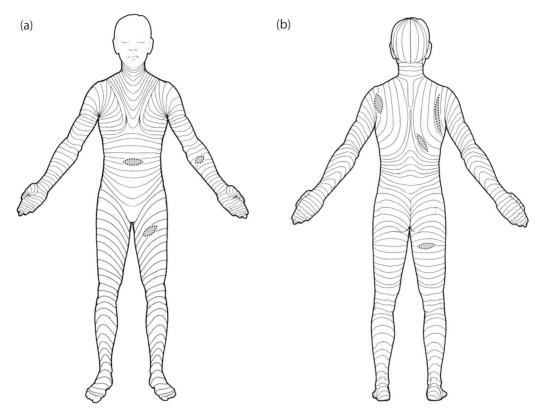

FIGURE 10.2 Maximum skin tension lines of trunk, extremities, scalp, and neck. (A) Anterior and (B) Posterior.

8. When stitching through the epidermal surface, the needle should enter the skin at a 90-degree angle (Figure 10.6 upper right).

    a. Rule of Halves: to minimize standing cones, place an epidermal suture in the middle first, then place second and third stiches on either side midway between the middle suture and the end of the excision closure, thereby dividing the linear closure into quarters (Figure 10.4A top).

    b. For wound closures with a lot of tension, more epidermal stitches can be placed in the central part of the closure than at the periphery.

9. Standing cones or "dog ears" are excess tissue that occurs at one end of the wound when wound edges are not the same length.

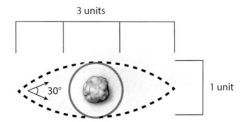

3 units

30°

1 unit

FIGURE 10.3 Ideal planned 3:1 fusiform excision with 30-degree angles at each apex.

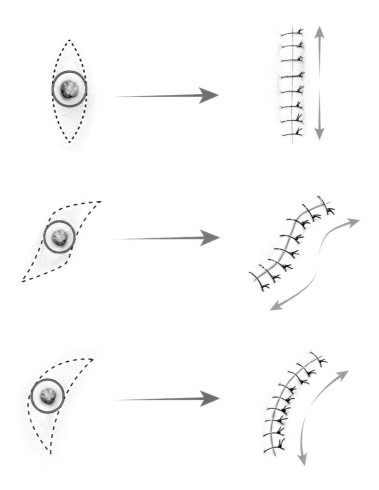

FIGURE 10.4 Different shaped excisions and their resultant closures. Top: fusiform excision. Middle: S-shaped excision used on convex or concave surfaces. Bottom: crescentic-shaped excision.

    a.   There are many ways to remove standing cones.

        i.   The most common technique involves making an incision straight through the center of the dog ear (Figure 10.7). Then the excess triangular skin on both sides of this incision is draped over the incision line and excised.

II. Basic Stitching Techniques: the basic principle that results in an imperceptible scar is close, even wound edge apposition with tensionless eversion. Epidermal wound edge tension can be minimized by placement of proper buried dermal/subcutaneous stitches. Epidermal/dermal stitches, cutaneous glue, tape, or staples can then be placed to produce and maintain epidermal approximation.[1–3]

    A. Buried stitches

        1. Interrupted buried stitches: useful for closing dead space, minimizing wound edge tension, and providing even wound edge apposition. Provides long-term dermal support during scar healing. Absorption time depends on suture type used.

            a.   The needle enters the subcutaneous tissue and exits the dermis, then reenters the opposite wound edge in the dermis where it courses inferiorly through the deep

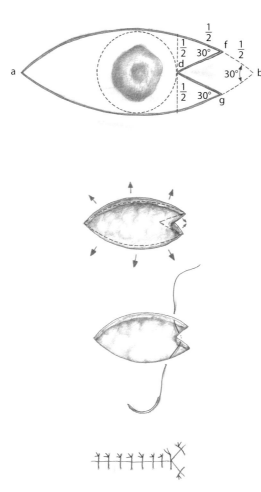

FIGURE 10.5 A M-plasty at one end of a fusiform excision. When healed, this geometric shape is harder to see than a straight line. Note that the M-plasty also shortens the fusiform excision. (Reproduced with permission from Bennett RG, *Fundamentals of Cutaneous Surgery*, C.V. Mosby, St. Louis, 1988.)

dermis and subcutaneous tissue; it then exits into the deep part of the wound. When the knot is tied, it is "buried" inside the wound below the dermis (Figure 10.8).

    b.   Important to place buried suture at same level on both sides of the wound to avoid a wound edge step-off.

  2. Purse string stitch: instead of vertical bites, this technique uses continuous horizontal bites in the deep dermis or subcutaneous tissue that, when cinched, partially or completely closes the wound depending on the wound size. If partially open, the remaining wound can be left to granulate or be grafted.

    a.   Useful in areas such as the lower leg or scalp where it is difficult to close a large wound side-to-side.

  3. Running dermal/subdermal stitch: this is a running buried stitch that is useful in wounds under mild tension.

B. Epidermal/dermal stitches: useful for producing wound edge eversion and close apposition, hemostasis, and decreasing wound edge tension. Can be used by itself as a top stitch in very low tension wounds, but otherwise used in combination with dermal/subcutaneous stitches.

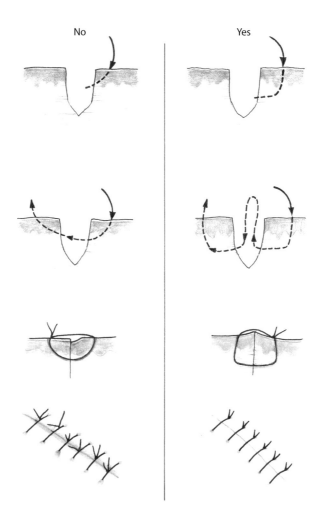

FIGURE 10.6 Interrupted epidermal/dermal stitch. Incorrect (left) and correct (right) suture path. Note on top right that suture enters skin at 90 degrees to skin surface and that on bottom right suture tails are pulled to one side of the wound. (Reproduced with permission from Bennett RG, *Fundamentals of Cutaneous Surgery*, C.V. Mosby, St. Louis, 1988.)

1. Interrupted stitch (Figure 10.6):
   a. On the face, enter 1–1.5 mm from the wound edge with the needle 90 degrees to the epidermis and come out through the dermis into the center of the incision with the needle, then enter at the same level of the dermis on the opposite wound edge and exit through the epidermis 1–1.5 mm from the wound edge. On the trunk and extremities, the suture needle enters and exits the skin about 2–2.5 mm from the wound edge.
   b. Care must be taken to enter and exit the epidermis at the same distance from the wound edge.
   c. Care must be taken to exit and enter both sides of the dermis at the same level to avoid a step off.
   d. Important to take a vertical bite of epidermis and dermis to allow for good eversion (Figure 10.6 top right).

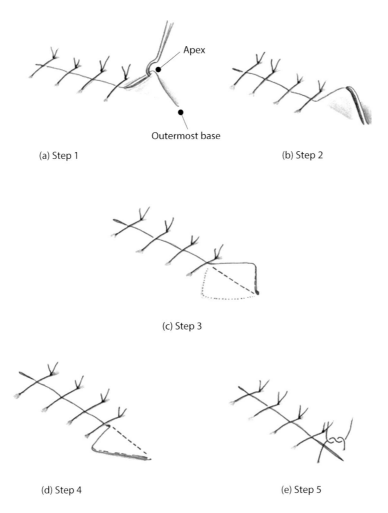

FIGURE 10.7 Dog ear (lying cone) excision that produces a straight line. (A) Step 1 Elevation of dog ear; (B) Step 2: A straight incision is made through the dog ear to its outermost base. This incision creates two equal triangles that are excised sequentially in Steps 3(C) and 4 (D). (E) Step 5 Suturing resultant straight line. (Reproduced with permission from Bennett RG, *Fundamentals of Cutaneous Surgery*, C.V. Mosby, St. Louis, 1988.)

2. Cutaneous running over-and-over stitch: a quicker stitch compared to simple interrupted stitches, useful in low tension areas (Figure 10.9).

   a. Similar technique to simple interrupted stitch, except that instead of tying off each knot and cutting the tails, this stitch is a continuously running over-and-over stitch that is tied off at each end. Compared to multiple interrupted stitches, the running over-and-over stitch results in more throws per unit length of wound and thus more complete wound apposition.

   b. Disadvantage is that if the stitch breaks, dehiscense can occur. To reduce the chance of dehiscense, an interrupted stitch can be placed in the center of the wound prior to placing the running over-and-over stitch.

   c. May scrunch wound edges if excision is curved.

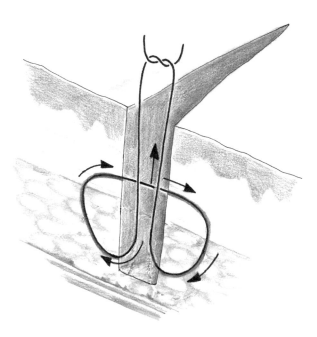

FIGURE 10.8   Buried dermal/subcutaneous stitch. Note that when the knot is tied, it is buried deep in the subcutaneous tissue. (Reproduced with permission from Bennett RG, *Fundamentals of Cutaneous Surgery*, C.V. Mosby, St. Louis, 1988.)

3. Running locked stitch: provides enhanced hemostasis. Useful in very vascular anatomic locations, such as the scalp, where there is an increased risk of blood flow and in high tension areas.
   a. Similar to a running over-and-over stitch, except the needle upon exiting the epidermis is passed under the preceding suture loop.

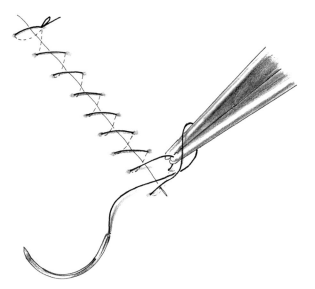

FIGURE 10.9   Running over-and-over stitch. (Reproduced with permission from Bennett RG, *Fundamentals of Cutaneous Surgery*, C.V. Mosby, St. Louis, 1988.)

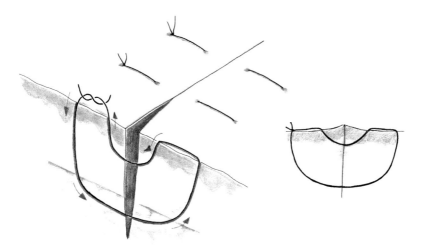

FIGURE 10.10   Vertical mattress (far far near near) stitch. (Reproduced with permission from Bennett RG, *Fundamentals of Cutaneous Surgery*, C.V. Mosby, St. Louis, 1988.)

4. Vertical mattress stitch (sometimes referred to as the "far far near near" stitch): this stitch is effective in everting the wound edges.

    a. The needle is introduced into the epidermis approximately 2–3 mm from the wound edge and passed through the wound to the opposite side where it exits the epidermis the same distance from the wound edge. The next entry point is into the epidermis from that same side in line with the previously placed suture about 1–1.5 mm from the wound edge; the needle then goes through the wound and exits the opposite epidermis the same distance from the wound edge. Then the suture is tied (Figure 10.10).

        i.   Be careful of tissue strangulation if suture pulled too tight.

        ii. There is also a running version of this stitch (the running vertical mattress stitch) that can be done or a vertical mattress stitch can be done as part of the running over-and-over stitch.

5. Horizontal mattress stitch: used for areas of high tension and also for hemostasis. Creates some eversion.

    a. The needle pierces the epidermis 2–3 mm from the wound edge, goes through the wound, and comes out on the opposite side the same distance from the wound edge. Then, 2–3 mm away from the wound edge on the same side and lateral and parallel to the wound edge, the needle pierces the epidermis; it then goes through the wound again, enters the opposite wound edge and exits the epidermis the same distance from and lateral to the original entrance point. Then it is tied.

        i.   As with the vertical mattress stitch, be careful to avoid tissue strangulation which might result in scarring.

6. Half-buried horizontal mattress stitch: also known as a tip stitch or 3-point stitch. This stitch creates close apposition of a triangular tip into an adjacent skin corner. This situation commonly occurs in a recipient skin flap wound.

    a. The needle enters the epidermis distal and slightly lateral to the recipient corner and exits the dermis into the wound (Figure 10.11 top). It then goes through the flap tip horizontally in the dermis, crosses the wound, and goes into the dermis on the opposite side of the wound. It then exits the epidermis at the same distance as the entrance point from the recipient corner but on the opposite side. The suture

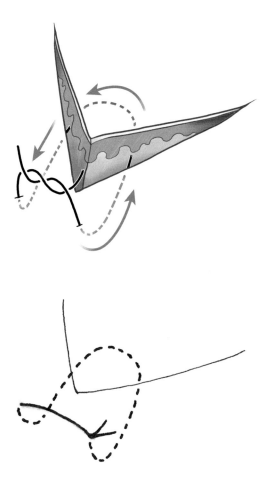

FIGURE 10.11 Half-buried horizontal mattress stitch. Note when tied (bottom) the knot is distal to the recipient corner. (Modified from Bennett RG, *Fundamentals of Cutaneous Surgery*, C.V. Mosby, St. Louis, 1988.)

is then tied. The knot should not be over the flap tip but more distal on the adjacent "receiving tissue" to avoid flap tip strangulation (Figure 10.11 bottom).

7. Running subcuticular or intradermal stitch: this stitch helps appose dermal and epidermal edges and prevents suture track marks.

    a. The needle pierces the epidermis 2–3 mm distal and slightly lateral to the future closure line. After emerging from the dermis into the wound, alternating horizontal dermal bites on either side of the wound edge are taken. Upon reaching the end of the sutured wound, the needle comes out through the dermis and epidermis about 2–3 mm distal and lateral to the closure line on the opposite side and end of the repair.

        i. The suture ends can be tied; however, this can result in tissue bunching.

        ii. The suture ends can also be taped.

        iii. The suture ends can also be buried after being tied.

        iv. Polypropylene is a good suture type to use with this stitch due to its low coefficient of friction allowing it to easily slip out of the tissue at the time of suture removal.

v. Of note, occasionally, the suture can get stuck during removal. To prevent this, a loop is created when suturing by coming through the epidermis in the center of the closure and then entering the epidermis on the opposite wound edge. When the loop is cut at the time of the suture removal, the length of the suture to be pulled out is halved with less likelihood of the suture getting hung up.

8. Pulley stitch – for wounds under extreme tension. This is the far-near near-far stitch that creates a loop within a loop. Thus, a pulley is created that when tied requires less force to close the wound.

9. Alternative methods for epidermal closure. Once the wound edges are tightly and evenly apposed with buried dermal/subdermal sutures, the following epidermal closure methods can be considered.

a. Tissue glue (e.g., Dermabond® [Ethicon], GluSeal® High Viscosity [GluStitch Inc.]).

b. Adhesive wound tape (e.g., Steri-Strips™ [3M]). Useful to reinforce wounds immediately after suture removal. Before application of wound tapes, a tackifier, such as tincture of benzoin or Mastisol® (Ferndale Laboratories, Inc. Ferndale, MI), is applied to the skin surface around a wound. If the wound tapes are kept dry they will stay in place for 5–7 days.

The main reason to wipe the skin surface with an antiseptic prior to excision is to remove transient bacterial pathogens.

c. Staples decrease risk of tissue strangulation because they do not completely envelop tissue as do stitches.

III. Additional Considerations for Excisional Surgery

A. Preoperative skin preparation

1. Prior to excisions and wound repairs, the surrounding skin is wiped or scrubbed with an antiseptic (Table 10.1). The main function of disinfectants is to remove transient bacterial pathogens from the skin surface.

2. Usually for skin surgery, either alcohol, povidone-iodine, or chlorhexidine is used. All are available in single-use packets.

TABLE 10.1

Antiseptic Surgical Scrubs

Agent (Product)	Antimicrobial Spectrum	Onset Time	Sustained Activity	Comments
70% isopropyl alcohol	Gram +, Gram -	Fastest	No	Antibacterial, does not kill spores, flammable
Tincture of Iodine, 2% free iodine + alcohol	Gram +, Gram -	Fast	Minimal	May sensitize patient, flammable
10% Povidone- iodine (e.g., Betadine®)	Gram +, Gram -	Moderate	Up to 1 hour	An iodofor (iodine + surfactant), must dry to be effective, activity enhanced if not removed, deactivated by blood
Chlorhexadine gluconate 4% (Hibiclens®)	Gram +, Gram -	Fast	Yes (hours)	Do not use around eyes or ears
Benzalkonium chloride 1% (Zephiran®)	Gram +, Gram -	Slow	No	Nonirritating to eyes

TABLE 10.2

Local Anesthetics (Injectable and Topical)

Chemical Name (Trade Name)	Onset	Duration	Amide or Ester	Maximum Dosage
Lidocaine (Xylocaine®)	15–30 min	1–2 hours with epinephrine	Amide	7 mg/kg with epinephrine and 4.5–5 mg/kg without epinephrine
Mepivacaine (Carbocaine®)	15–30 min	1–2 hours with epinephrine	Amide	7 mg/kg
Bupivacaine (Marcaine®)	30–45 min	4–6 hours with epinephrine	Amide	2.5 mg/kg
Lidocaine 4% cream (ELA-Max, LMX4®) lidocaine 5% cream (LMX5®)	5–10 min (eyelids, genitalia)[b]	1 hour	Amide	Topical (skin) Adult: 400 cm² skin surface area
Lidocaine 2.5%/ prilocaine 2.5% cream (EMLA)	5–10 min (eyelids, genitalia)[b]	1 hour	Amide	Topical (skin) Adult: 3 mg/kg Infant: 1–2 g[c] Child: 10–20 g[c]
Procaine[a] (Novocaine®)	2–5 min	30–60 min	Ester	15 mg/kg
Proparacaine (Alcaine®)	30 sec	5–10 min	Ester	Topical (cornea/ conjunctiva)
Tetracaine (Pontocaine®)	30 sec	10 min	Ester	Topical (0.5% cornea/ conjunctiva, 2–4% skin)
Benzocaine	5–10 min	1 hour	Ester	Topical (5%, 20% skin)

[a] Not used in dermatology.
[b] 30 min with occlusion elsewhere.
[c] One fingertip unit = 0.5 g.

   3. Chlorohexidine should not be used around the eyes or ears as it can damage the cornea and be ototoxic.
   4. Benzalkonium chloride is useful around the eyes.

  B. Local anesthetics

   1. Mechanism of action: reversibly inhibit nerve conduction by blocking sodium ion influx into nerve cells. Thus, local anesthetics prevent nerve depolarization.
   2. The commonly used local anesthetics are shown in Table 10.2.
   3. The most common local anesthetic used is lidocaine 1% (10 mg/cc) with epinephrine 1:100,000 units. The maximum safe dose in adults with this concentration is about 30–40 cc infiltrated into skin. Specifically, the maximum recommended dose is 7 mg/kg (or 4.5 mg/kg if without epinephrine). For a typical 70 kg adult, this computes into approximately 50 cc with epinephrine (or 32 cc without epinephrine). The $T_{1/2}$ is about 90 minutes. However, since lidocaine is metabolized in the liver by microsomal enzymes (cytochrome p450 3A4) and excreted by the kidneys, caution is required for patients with liver or renal disease.
   4. A 30-gauge needle is typically used for injection to decrease pain.
   5. The slower the injection rate, the less pain the patient will experience.
   6. Lidocaine allergy is rare. If a patient states they are allergic to lidocaine, mepivacaine or bupivacaine may be possible to use because usually patients don't cross react. Usually allergic lidocaine reactions are due to para-aminobenzoic acid (PABA) used as a preservative in anesthetic solutions. Therefore, preservative-free lidocaine, mepivacaine, or bupivacaine can be used if patient is PABA sensitive. Another alternative

TABLE 10.3

Commonly Used Absorbable Sutures

Material	Configuration	Time to Absorption (Days)	Brand Name
Plain Gut[b]	Multifilament twisted	70	Same as generic
Fast Absorbing Gut[b]	Multifilament twisted	21–42	Same as generic
Chromic Gut[b]	Multifilament twisted	90	Same as generic
Polyglycolic Acid[c]	Multifilament braided	60–90	Dexon™
Polyglactin 910[a,c]	Multifilament braided	56–70	Vicryl™
Polydioxanone[a,c]	Monofilament	90–180	PDS®
Glycolide and polytrimethylene carbonate[a]	Monofilament	60–180	Maxon™
Poliglecaprone 25[c]	Monofilament	90–120	Monocryl®
Glycomer 631[c]	Monofilament	100	Biosyn™

[a] Also available as "Plus" with antibacterial triclosan.
[b] Gut made from sheep or beef intestinal submucosa. Degraded by proteolysis.
[c] Synthetic, degraded by hydrolysis.

local anesthetic would be diphenhydramine (Benadryl®) solution which comes in bottles at a concentration of 50 mg/cc. Although diphenhydramine works well for providing local anesthesia, because of its sedative effects, one has to be mindful of the total dose.

7. For patients who complain of reactions to epinephrine (sweating, palpitations), or have a history of hypertension or heart problems (arrhythmias, myocardial infarction), one can use a local anesthetic without epinephrine or with a lesser epinephrine concentration (1:200,000). The lesser epinephrine concentration still achieves adequate hemostasis.

8. Topical anesthetic creams are sometimes used alone or prior to local anesthetic injections. However, these creams are most effective on the eyelids or genitalia where the dermis is thin.

C. Suture properties – sutures are classified into two categories: absorbable (Table 10.3) and nonabsorbable (Table 10.4).[4]

1. Physical properties of sutures: determines handling, stability, and ease of tying knots.
   a. Configuration:
      i. Monofilament.
      ii. Multifilament: twisted or braided.
         a) Silk is a soft braided suture useful in mucosal surfaces or the genitalia where it does not irritate the patient.

TABLE 10.4

Commonly Used Nonabsorbable Sutures

Suture	Configuration	Brand Name
Silk	Multifilament braided	Same as generic
Nylon	Monofilament	Ethilon®, Dermalon™
Polypropylene	Monofilament	Prolene®, Surgilene®
Polyester	Multifilament Braided	Mersilene®
Polybutester	Monofilament	Novafil™

        b) Polyglactin 910 or polyglycolic acid are braided sutures that are easy to tie and handle and used most often for dermal/subdermal stitches.

        c) Advantages: increased tensile strength, improved handling, improved knot tying.

        d) Disadvantages: increased resistance when pulled through tissue, increased risk of infection from microorganisms that can lodge and proliferate within the interstices of the multiple twists or braids.

b. Coefficient of friction: determines how easily suture will pass through skin.

   i. A low coefficient of friction implies it is easy to pull suture through skin.

   ii. Sutures with a low coefficient of friction may require more throws for knot security because they are usually more slippery.

   iii. Polypropylene is an example of a nonabsorbable suture with a very low coefficient of friction.

c. Coating: lowers the coefficient of friction of a material.

   i. Silicone, Teflon™ (DuPont, Wilmington, DE), wax, antibacterial agents.

d. Capillarity: ability of fluids to pass from moist end to dry end.

   i. Braided sutures have increased capillarity and may suck in and thus harbor bacteria along with moisture or fluid.

e. Tensile strength: weight needed to break a suture as a function of its cross-sectional area or diameter.

   i. Multifilament > Monofilament.

   ii. Synthetic > Natural.

   iii. Surgical stainless steel sutures have the highest tensile strength.

f. Suture diameter (caliber).

   i. The greater the diameter, the greater the tensile strength.

   ii. The smaller the number before the "0" size the larger the diameter. (Thus, the 3–0 suture has a larger diameter than a 6–0 suture.) The "0" is pronounced as the letter "O" not the numerical zero.

> Small diameter sutures are more likely to tear through tissue than large diameter sutures.

   iii. The smaller the suture diameter, the more likely it is to tear or cut through tissue than suture with a larger diameter.

g. Knot strength: determined by the force needed to cause a knot to slip.

   i. Increased coefficient of friction improves knot strength.

h. Memory: ability of suture to retain its original straight shape after being bent.

   i. Sutures with increased memory are more difficult to handle and are prone to unraveling as the suture will try to revert to its original (straight) configuration.

i. Elasticity: ability of suture to return to original form and length after being stretched.

   i. If swelling occurs at the suture site, sutures with elastic properties can swell with the wound and are thus less likely to cause stitch marks.

j. Plasticity: ability of suture to retain distortion once it is stretched with no ability to regain original form.

   i. Polypropylene exhibits plasticity.

      ii.   Will stretch to accommodate edema, but suture will lose ability to evert skin due to weaker ability to properly oppose tissue once swelling subsides.

      iii. Rarely produces "stitch marks" as it stretches with wound edema.

Polypropylene sutures are usually used to suture skin edges together as they rarely produce suture track marks.

   k. Tissue reactivity: the tissue inflammatory response elicited by sutures; determined by various suture properties.

      i.   Large diameter > Small diameter.

      ii. Natural > Synthetic.

      iii. Absorbable > Nonabsorbable.

      iv. Multifilament > Monofilament.

   l. Absorption: ability of suture material to lose most of its tensile strength by degradation.

      i.   Absorbable sutures lose most of their tensile strength by 60 days. Catgut usually absorbs by 60 days. Polyglactin usually absorbs by 90 days.

      ii. Nonabsorbable sutures take much longer than 60 days. Sometimes absorption may take years.

      iii. Animal-derived sutures (gut) are broken down by proteolysis and then absorbed, whereas synthetic sutures are broken down slowly by hydrolysis.

      iv. Absorption altered by presence of infection, suture type, and site of suture placement.

D. Needle properties

   1. Composed of three parts (Figure 10.12):

     a. Shank: portion that attaches to suture, weakest part of needle.

     b. Body: strongest part of needle. The jaw tips of the needle holder should grasp the body in the center, especially if the needle is delicate, to keep it from bending during placement.

     c. Point: includes the needle tip.

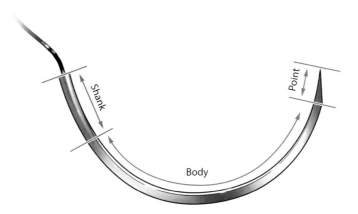

FIGURE 10.12   Parts of the surgical needle. (Modified from Bennett RG, *Fundamentals of Cutaneous Surgery*, C.V. Mosby, St. Louis, 1988.)

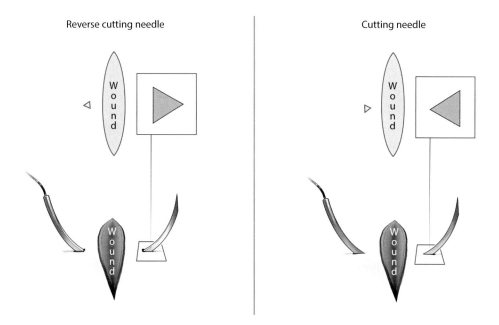

FIGURE 10.13 Needle wounds due to distal needle body shape that is triangular on cross-section. (Left) Reverse cutting. (Right) Conventional cutting. Note greater tendency of suture to tear or cut tissue with conventional cutting needle compared to reverse cutting needle.

2. Variety of needles.
   a. Can be straight or curved (latter most commonly used by dermatologic surgeons).
      i. Curvature of 3/8 circle is most commonly used.
      ii. Also available: 1/4, 1/2, 3/4, 5/8 circle curvatures.
   b. Types: based on cross-section shape of the distal needle body (Figure 10.13):
      i. Round: produces least amount of tissue tearing, useful for suturing tendons.
      ii. Conventional cutting: the distal needle body is triangular on cross-section with one triangle corner on the inside and one flat triangle side on the outside of the needle. Therefore, when going through epidermis the cutting edge is closest to wound edge resulting in potential tissue tearing by suture.

      > The cost of sutures is related more to the needle type than the suture material.

      iii. Reverse cutting: the distal needle body is triangular on cross-section with one triangle corner tip on the outside and one flat triangle side on the inside of the needle. Therefore, when going through epidermis, the cutting edge is away from the wound edge and thus suture is less likely to tear tissue than suture on the conventional cutting needle. The reverse cutting needle is most commonly used in skin surgery.

IV. Postoperative Wound Care
   A. Dressings: initially, the following is placed on the wound (see Figure 9.1).
      1. Antibiotic ointment (Table 10.1). Generally, we use Polysporin® (polymyxin B sulfate/bacitracin) ointment because it is sterile, spreads easily, and has a low sensitization rate. An alternative for patients sensitive to antibiotic containing ointments is Vaseline® (white petrolatum).

    2. Nonstick dressing material (e.g., Telfa™ [Smith & Nephew])

    3. Gauze

    4. Paper tape (usually Micropore Flesh Tone® 3M)

B. At the time of the first dressing change (usually 24 hours later), the wound is cleansed with 3% hydrogen peroxide or 0.9 % normal saline solution and a new dressing is applied using:

    1. Antibiotic ointment.

    2. Nonstick dressing material. Usually additional gauze is not necessary.

    3. Paper tape.

C. Dressings are changed daily until suture removal.

D. Patients can get their wounds wet after 24 hours. If the patient showers with the dressing on, he or she should change it immediately afterwards to keep the wound from becoming macerated.

E. Avoid swimming or exercise that puts tension on the sutured wound until 1–2 weeks after suture removal.

F. Suture removal: sutures are generally removed in 7–10 days. Sutures are left longer (14–21 days) on trunk, extremities, and scalp. Modern sutures, especially polypropylene, can be left in place for long periods of time without causing suture track marks. After suture removal, a tacky liquid adhesive, such as Mastisol® (Ferndale Laboratories, Ferndale, MI), is applied around the wound and adhesive strips, such as Steri-Strips™ (3M, Maplewood, MN), are applied across the wound to bolster the healing wound. If the area is kept dry, the Steri-Strips will stay on up to 1–2 weeks.

V. Complications

A. Infection – can be minimized by disinfecting skin on excision site prior to excision to remove transient pathogens. Most commonly used is alcohol wipes, povidone-iodine, or chlorhexidine (Table 10.1).

    1. Should the sutured wound appear infected (redness, pain, pus) a culture should be done. Appropriate antibiotics should be given.

    2. Topical solutions that may be considered to treat open infected wounds are shown in Table 10.5; topical antibiotic ointments and creams are shown in Table 10.1.

B. Bleeding (hematoma) – can be minimized by careful hemostasis prior to wound closure.

C. Dehiscence – avoided by taking tension off wound edges at time of closure. Also minimized by patient avoiding heavy lifting, stretching, and walking (if on the lower leg or foot) in the immediate postoperative period for 1–2 weeks. May result in depressed or spread scars.

TABLE 10.5

Useful Topical Solutions for Infected Wounds

Name	Active Component	Spectrum of Activity	Preparations
White vinegar solution	Acetic acid	Pseudomonas	One part vinegar to three parts water
Acetic acid solution	Acetic acid	Pseudomonas	1–5% solution
Silver nitrate solution	Silver nitrate	Gram -	0.25–0.5% aqueous solution
Dakin's solution	Sodium hypochlorite	Gram +, Gram -	Solution 0.5%
Burow's solution	Aluminum acetate	Gram +	Solution 1:40 (1 Domeboro tablet in a pint of tap water)
Potassium permanganate solution	Potassium permanganate	Gram +, Gram -	1:10,000

D. Skin necrosis – due to excess tension or inadequate blood supply. Treat by keeping wound moist and covered until healed. Minimize tobacco use.

E. Spitting sutures – if buried dermal/subdermal sutures and/or their suture tails are close to wound surface, these sutures may partially or completely extrude. Usually these buried sutures are removed when the patient returns for his or her follow-up visit.

F. Contact dermatitis – can occur with prolonged use of any antibacterial ointment, but especially neomycin. Appears as pruritic poorly defined erythemtous area of skin surrounding wound. Treat by having patient use white petrolatum (Vaseline®) on the wound. If extensive and very pruritic, may need to prescribe a topical corticosteroid ointment (e.g., triamcinolone acetonide ointment 0.1%) to be used on red area around wound twice a day.

G. Allergy to suture – very rare with synthetic sutures. However, allergic reaction to catgut can occur if patient is sensitive to beef.

H. Foreign body reaction to sutures.

I. Suture track marks – unusual with polypropylene sutures but more common with nylon. May be related to delayed suture removal but more likely to sutures being tied too tight. Suture track marks can be improved with dermabrasion or laser.

J. Keloids/hypertrophic scars – often anatomically dependent; common on upper trunk. If these occur, may improve with intralesional injection of triamcinolone acetonide (Kenalog®-10). Injections may be repeated every 4 weeks.

K. Hyperpigmentation of healed scar – can occur in darker skin patients with sun exposure. Can be avoided by use of broad spectrum sunscreens after surgery. Treated by chemical peel, laser, or hydroquinone cream.

L. Hypopigmentation of scar – often shows up in contrast to surrounding erythema. Treated by decreasing surrounding erythema with laser or tattooing scar with pigment to match the surrounding skin color.

Conclusion

Mastery of fundamental excision technique and various stitch and suture types will result in an optimal functional and cosmetic outcome.

REFERENCES

1. Bennett RG. Fundamentals of Cutaneous Surgery. C.V. Mosby Company, St. Louis, Missouri, 1988; pp. 179–491.
2. Moy RL, Waldman B, Hein DW. A Review of Sutures and Suturing Techniques. J Dermatol Surg Oncol 1992; 18: 785–795.
3. Weitzl S, Taylor RS. Suturing techniques and other closure materials. In: Surgery of the Skin: Procedural Dermatology. 2nd Edition (Robinson JK, Hanke CW, Siegel DM, Fratila A, editors). Mosby Elsevier, New York, NY, 2010; pp. 189–209.
4. Bennett RG. Selection of Wound Closure Materials. J Am Acad Dermatol 1988; 18: 619–637.

11

Nail Unit Surgery

Michael Xiong and Richard G. Bennett

Introduction

Nail unit surgery requires anatomic knowledge of the nail and its close connection to surrounding structures. Understanding this adnexal relationship will assist the physician in selecting a procedure that will result in the greatest likelihood of diagnosis and cure for a nail problem while providing the optimal functional and cosmetic result.

I. Anatomy (Figures 11.1A and B)
- A. Nail
    1. Slightly curved convex plate composed of hard compact keratin.
    2. Covers and protects dorsal distal digit.
    3. Helps gripping and scratching.
    4. Has cosmetic value, especially for women.
    5. Extends from matrix proximally (from which it is derived) to distal groove distally.
    6. The nail plate is thinnest over the matrix.
    7. Develops in embryo beginning at weeks 9–10 for fingernails and weeks 15–16 for toenails.[1]
    8. Grows at rate of 3 mm/month for fingernails and 1 mm/month for toenails. Fingernails regrow in 4–6 months, whereas toenails regrow in 12–18 months.[1]

    > Nails grow very slowly. It takes 4–6 months for fingernails and 12–18 months for toenails to regrow.

- B. Nail matrix
    1. Generates the nail plate. Nail growth rate correlates to matrix cell turnover.
    2. Lacks a granular layer. Contains melanocytes, most prominent in distal matrix.[1] Also contains Langerhans and Merkel cells.
    3. Lies beneath the proximal nail plate above the mid portion of the distal phalanx and extends to the nail bed. Its proximal edge is just distal to the insertion of the extensor tendon. The distal matrix can be seen through the nail plate as a white crescent-shaped structure called the lunula (a diminutive of the Latin word *luna* meaning moon). The lunula is most prominent under the thumbnail and first toenail.
    4. The matrix shape is shown in Figure 11.1A. Note on the median and lateral side the matrix comes to an acute angle. This pointed area is known as the horn. The horn becomes important when excising the matrix because if it is overlooked and left intact, this small remaining portion of the matrix will produce a nail spicule. This spicule is annoying and on the finger can catch when placing one's hand in a pocket.

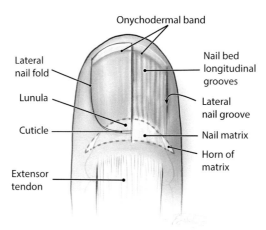

FIGURE 11.1A Nail and its adnexa – dorsal view.

5. Top and bottom of nail plate generated by different areas of matrix.
    a. Proximal matrix generates the dorsal portion of the nail plate. Disruption of the proximal matrix leads to a superficial defect in the nail plate resulting in onychorrhexis (superficial horizontal nail fragmentation) or onychoschizia (both horizontal and/or longitudinal nail breakage) (Table 11.1).

    > Proximal matrix generates dorsal nail plate. Distal matrix generates ventral nail plate.

    b. Distal matrix generates the ventral portion of the nail plate. Disruption of distal matrix (e.g., surgery, neoplasm) → defect of ventral nail plate, resulting in longitudinal erythronychia or onychomadesis (separation of nail plate from proximal nail bed and/or matrix).
6. Extensor tendon inserts on dorsal distal phalanx bone usually 10–12 mm proximal to cuticle. This location is just proximal to the nail matrix near its midline.
C. Nail bed
    1. Supports nail plate.
    2. Extends from distal matrix to distal groove.
    3. The nail bed epidermis fits into dermal longitudinal grooves. This tongue-in-groove arrangement appears as regularly aligned longitudinal epidermal ridges and dermal grooves that provide strong adhesion of the nail plate to the nail bed. The grooves also provide directionality to nail growth. As the nail plate thins in old age, the underlying grooves become visible.
        a. Onycholysis – distal separation of nail plate from nail bed. Nail appears clear.
        b. Onychomadesis – proximal separation of the nail plate from the nail bed and/or matrix.
    4. Appears reddish in color due to the rich blood supply.
    5. Does not contain subcutaneous tissue. Nail bed dermis attaches directly onto underlying periosteum.
D. Distal nail structures (Figure 11.1B)
    1. Most inferiorly – the hyponychium. A thickened (acanthotic) distal extension of the nail bed epidermis that becomes contiguous more distally with the digit epidermis. Has a granular layer; the only part of the nail unit with a granular layer and the first

TABLE 11.1

Onycho Whatever

Onychatrophy (onychatrophia)	Defective development of nail
Onychalgia	Nail unit pain
Onychochauxis	Abnormally thickened nail
Onychochasis	Breaking of nail
Onychocryptosis	Ingrown nail
Onychodystrophy	Malformation of nail
Onychogryphosis	Curvature and horn-like hypertrophy of nail
Onychoheterotopia	Abnormally placed nail on bed as a result of displaced matrix
Onychia	A pathologic condition or inflammation somewhere in the nail unit, often the matrix
Onycholysis	Distal separation of nail plate from nail bed
Onychomadesis	Separation of nail from proximal nail bed and/or matrix. Results in loss of nail
Onychomalacia	Softened nail
Onychomycosis	Fungal infection of nail
Onychopathy	Disease of the nails
Onychophyma	Onychochauxis
Onychoptosis	Loss of nail plate
Onychoschizia	Distal horizontal and/or longitudinal nail splitting
Onychorrhexis	Superficial horizontal nail plate fragmentation
Onychosis	Disease of the nails

site of increased keratinization of the nail unit. The gradual thickened nail bed epidermis and keratin produced forms the onychodermal band (see below).

2. The distal groove – lies distal to the hyponychium. Separates hyponychium from distal nail fold and digit epidermis.

3. Onychodermal band – a band visible just proximal to the distal white-free edge of the nail. It represents thickened nail bed epidermis and keratin proliferation from the hyponychium below the distal nail plate. This thickened keratin is attached tightly to the inferior distal nail plate. It forms a seal between the nail plate and the hyponychium. Thus, the onychodermal band helps prevent onycholysis subsequent to trauma. The keratotic distal end of the onychodermal band under the free nail plate edge is known as the solehorn.

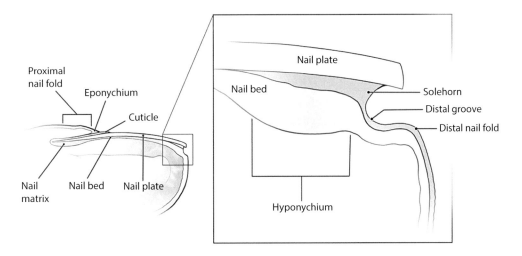

FIGURE 11.1B Nail and its adnexa – lateral view.

E. Proximal nail fold
   1. Covers and protects proximal newly formed nail plate and its underlying matrix.
   2. Has a dorsal and ventral surface seen on cross-section.
   3. Cuticle – thin web-shaped keratotic extension onto the nail surface from the ventral proximal nail fold. Seals and protects nail from outside pathogens. If injured, may lead to bacterial infection underneath the nail folds (paronychia).
   4. Eponychium – thin portion of proximal nail fold just proximal to cuticle. Represents the junction of the dorsal and ventral epidermal surface of the proximal nail fold. In some textbooks eponychium is synonymous with cuticle, whereas other textbooks distinguish these two entities.

F. Lateral nail fold
   1. Rolled skin that protects and cushions the lateral nail plate on either side.
   2. Forms a groove between itself and the nail bed.
   3. Contiguous with the proximal nail fold and the distal nail fold.

II. Anesthesia
   A. Local infiltrative anesthesia
      1. Generally avoided as a primary method of anesthesia around the nail plate because in this area skin is tight and thus very painful when anesthetic is injected into the tight space.
   B. Digital nerve block
      1. Use 2% lidocaine without epinephrine. 2% lidocaine is used in all nerve blocks because the high concentration of anesthetic diffuses across nerve membranes more readily than lower concentrations (e.g., 1% lidocaine).
      2. Epinephrine is not used in digital nerve blocks because on the toes necrosis can occur with underlying diabetes or peripheral vascular disease.
      3. The dorsal and ventral digital nerves run longitudinally along the length of the digits. To adequately anesthetize these nerves enough length of these nerves must be exposed to anesthetic solution. Thus we inject proximally and distally in addition to superiorly and inferiorly on both sides of the digit between the proximal interphalangeal joint and the metacarpophalangeal or metatarsophalangeal joint as shown in Figure 11.2.

      > Use 2% lidocaine for digital nerve block anesthesia.

      4. Need to wait 15 minutes for nerve block anesthesia to take effect. Better more numb than quick.
      5. Occasionally needs to be supplemented by infiltration on either side of proximal nail fold, known as "wing block". Usually this is not necessary unless digital nerve block is inadequate because of insufficient anesthetic solution, its poor placement, or not waiting an adequate period of time (usually 15 minutes).
      6. Avoid a ring block infiltrating anesthetic around the whole digit. Doing so may produce a "fluid tourniquet".

III. Instruments
   A. Nail elevator
      1. A Freer elevator has flat spatula-like surface that allows it to be easily inserted between nail plate and its bed to atraumatically detach the nail plate.
   B. Nail nipper
      1. Thick jaws allow cutting of very thick nail plate.

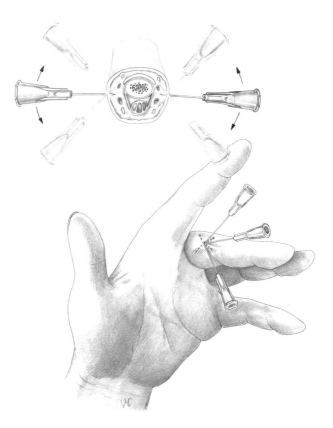

FIGURE 11.2   Digital nerve block. (Reproduced with permission from Bennett RG, *Fundamentals of Cutaneous Surgery*, C.V. Mosby, St. Louis, 1988.)

    C. Nail splitter (Figure 11.3)
        1. One jaw blade is flattened on its outside edge to glide atraumatically between nail bed and nail plate. The other jaw has a rounded end so that it pushes against rather than through the proximal nail fold.
        2. An essential instrument for nail surgery.

IV. Hemostasis
    A. Surgery on the end of the digits is usually bloody, especially since a nerve block is usually done with 2% lidocaine without epinephrine. Lidocaine is itself a vasodilator.
    B. A sterile glove may be used to provide hemostasis and at the same time to exsanguinate blood from the digit (Figure 11.4). The glove is fitted over the patient's hand after which the glove fingertip is cut off. Then the remaining glove finger is rolled on itself proximally which gradually tightens to provide a tourniquet effect at the finger base. The remainder of the glove is kept in place to provide a sterile field.
        1. The sterile glove technique works well on the hand. On the foot it is only useful on the first toe.
    C. A ½ or 1 inch Penrose drain is useful to provide a tourniquet during surgery.
        1. The broad width of the Penrose drain avoids tissue necrosis and vasospasm that could occur with narrow tourniquets, such as a rubber band.
        2. The Penrose drain is placed around the finger or toe and secured with a hemostat (Figure 11.5). The hemostat is then rotated in a circle 2 or 3 times to tighten the

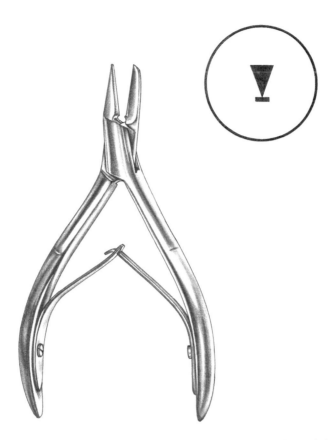

FIGURE 11.3 Nail splitter with cross-section through tip (inset). (Reproduced with permission from Bennett RG, *Fundamentals of Cutaneous Surgery*, C.V. Mosby, St. Louis, 1988.)

Penrose drain. This technique requires an assistant to hold the hemostat in place during surgery. The blood flow to the fingertip can be adjusted by the number of turns of the hemostat.

To avoid vasospasm and necrosis, a Penrose drain is recommended as a finger or toe tourniquet.

3. There have been instances where a patient has left a physician's office with a rubber band tourniquet in place resulting in finger necrosis. With a Penrose drain and hemostat, this situation would be unlikely.

D. Tourniquet time. Most nail procedures last from a few minutes to half an hour. A tourniquet can safely be left in place for this period of time. For longer procedures, the tourniquet may be loosened temporarily for 10 minutes to allow blood flow and then reapplied. It is a good idea to record the total time the tourniquet is in place (the "tourniquet time").

V. Disinfection

A. Surgical wounds on the digits can become infected because the blood supply in this area is less than in other areas of the body, particularly in the elderly.

B. Disinfection is done prior to surgery on the nail and its adnexa. We use povidone-iodine swabsticks (Dynarex Corporation, Orangeburg, NY) or chlorhexidine gluconate swabsticks (Hibiclens, Prevantics, Woodcliff Lakes, NJ).

C. Preoperative and postoperative antibiotics may be considered especially when operating on inflamed periungual tissues such as ingrown nails.

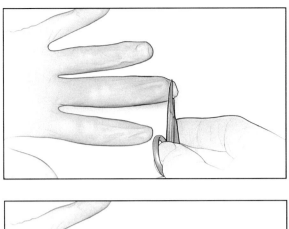

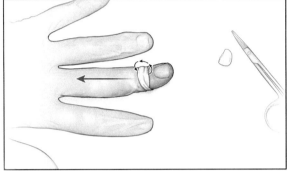

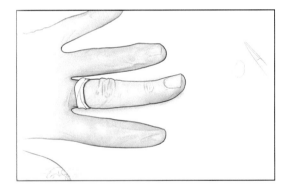

FIGURE 11.4   Sterile glove used to create tourniquet.

VI. Surgical techniques to gain exposure under nail and proximal nail fold
    A. Nail removal (avulsion)
        1. Nail is removed by its separation from nail bed, matrix and nail folds, lateral and proximal. May be partial for localized lesions under nail plate.
        2. Useful to soak nail in water for 20 minutes prior to avulsion. This soaking helps to soften nail and facilitates cutting through it.
        3. Use nail elevator to detach nail. Its thin flat surface is inserted under the distal nail and pushed proximally and side-to-side laterally. Then a hemostat pulls the nail free.
        4. If the proximal nail fold is adherent to the nail, the nail elevator may be inserted under the nail fold to separate it from the underlying nail prior to nail avulsion.

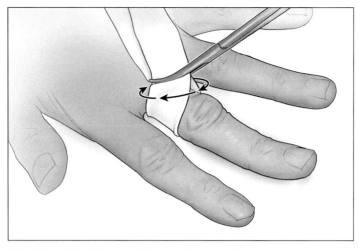

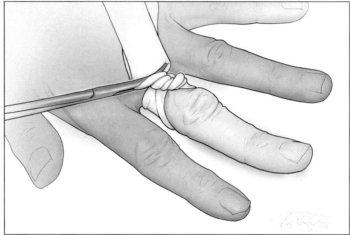

FIGURE 11.5   Penrose drain used to create digital tourniquet.

5. An alternative method to remove a nail plate is to use the nail splitter to split the nail plate in two. Then grasp one half of the nail plate with a hemostat and twist until separation occurs. Repeat on the remaining half of the nail if necessary to remove the whole nail.

6. The nail bed epidermis is tightly adherent to the nail and comes off with the avulsed nail.

B. Proximal nail fold reflection (Figure 11.6)

1. Useful to expose entire matrix or to access growths under proximal nail fold.

2. Two oblique incisions made on either side of proximal nail fold. The proximal nail fold is freed from the underlying nail with blunt tipped tenotomy scissors or a Freer elevator.

3. The proximal nail fold is reflected proximally using two skin hooks.

4. After whatever procedure has been completed underneath the reflected posterior nail fold, it is stitched back into place.

5. We place the first suture at the junction of the distal oblique cut edge and the lateral nail fold so as to line up exactly the junction of the proximal and lateral nail folds.

6. Remaining interrupted stitches are then placed.

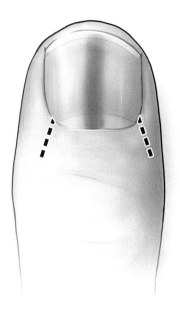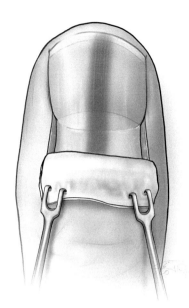

FIGURE 11.6 Reflection back of proximal nail fold.

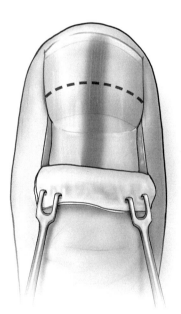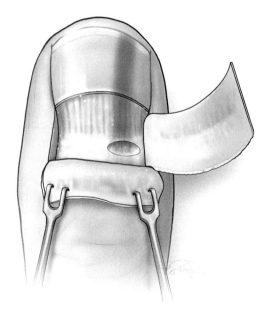

FIGURE 11.7 Reflection back of proximal nail fold with proximal nail reflection.

C. Partial proximal nail plate reflection[3] (Figure 11.7)

1. Useful to expose nail bed and matrix proximally and still retain complete nail.

2. The posterior nail fold is reflected back by two oblique incisions (see Figure 11.5).

3. The nail is then transversely cut by an incision across the proximal one-third to one-half of the nail plate. This cut is made by a nail splitter that is inserted transversely into one lateral nail sulcus.

TABLE 11.2

Nail Biopsy and Excision Techniques

Technique	Uses	Advantages	Disadvantages
Double Punch Biopsy	Pigmented lesion <3 mm	Quick. No whole or partial nail plate removal necessary.	Small sample size. May require reflection proximal nail fold. Risk of nail dystrophy if done on proximal matrix.
Shave Biopsy	Pigmented lesion >3 mm	Useful for broad lesion on nail bed or matrix. Adequate sample. Heals by granulation.	Partial nail plate reflection or partial or complete avulsion necessary.
Small Excision	Small lesions <3 mm	May be sutured for fast healing. Complete removal.	Partial nail plate reflection or partial or complete avulsion necessary. If involves matrix, may result in nail dystrophy.
Lateral Longitudinal Excision	1. Ingrown nail. 2. Atypical pigmented lesion adjacent to lateral nail fold. 3. To diagnose nail dermatologic disease associated with nail (i.e., psoriasis).	Adequate sample of complete nail unit.	Permanently narrow nail plate. If matrix horn not removed, nail spicule may appear near lateral end of proximal nail fold. Postoperative pain.
Median Longitudinal Excision	Atypical pigmented lesion in mid-nail.	Adequate sample of complete nail unit.	Nail dystrophy (onychoschizia). Permanently narrow nail plate. Postoperative pain.

4. The transverse cut starts from one nail edge and extends toward the opposite nail edge where a small amount of nail plate is left intact.

5. The proximal nail is then freed up and reflected back with a hemostat to one side exposing the nail bed and nail matrix. The distal nail plate remains in place. Thus, this is similar to opening the top of a dutch door.

6. After the matrix biopsy or excision is performed, the nail plate is put back in place. A small amount of free lateral nail edge is trimmed longitudinally by 2–3 mm to reduce postoperative pain and swelling prior to replacement into the lateral nail fold.

7. The proximal nail fold is put into place and sutured.

8. The nail plate is sutured to the lateral nail fold.[3]

VII. Biopsy and Small Excision Techniques (Table 11.2)

A. Double punch biopsy through nail plate (Figure 11.8)

The "double punch" technique is suggested to biopsy through the nail plate.

1. Useful for lesions of the nail bed or nail matrix.

2. Quick.

3. Does not require removal of nail plate, but for exposure of full matrix may require reflection of proximal nail fold.

4. Two punches are used (usually a 3 mm and 4 mm). The larger 4 mm punch goes only through the nail plate. One first scores the nail with the 4 mm punch to ascertain that one is in the precise location before going deeper and through the nail.[4] The punch is then returned to the scored nail and turned to go completely through the nail plate which is removed. Be aware that oftentimes the removed nail plate is lodged in the

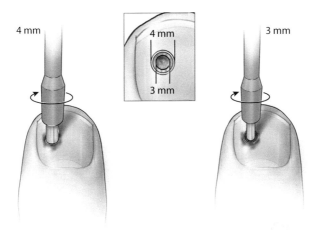

FIGURE 11.8   Double punch technique. 4 mm punch (Left) used first to remove nail plate only. 3 mm punch (Right) used to remove nail bed to bone.

punch.[2] Then the smaller 3 mm punch is used to remove underlying nail bed tissue. Depth of second punch usually to bone.

5. Handle nail bed tissue with delicate instruments; avoid crushing tissue. Usually to remove the punch biopsy from nail bed, a scalpel blade tip is used to dissect the punch-cut nail bed from underlying bone.

6. Bleeding is stopped with pressure. Do not apply Monsel solution (Ferric subsulfate) as iron pigment in tissue can be confused with melanoma pigment if a subsequent melanoma excision is necessary.

7. Drawback may be not obtaining an adequate sample.

B. Punch biopsy after reflecting back posterior nail fold with and without nail plate avulsion (Figure 11.9).

1. To gain access to the matrix underlying the posterior nail fold, two oblique incisions are made on either side of the posterior nail fold. The nail fold is then undermined gently and reflected back proximally. This maneuver exposes the underlying nail plate beneath which is the matrix.

2. Because the nail plate is thin and soft in this area, either a single punch biopsy or double punch biopsy can be performed.

3. A punch into distal matrix may not result in significant nail deformity; however, a punch into proximal matrix will result in permanent nail deformity.[3]

4. A punch greater than 3 mm is more likely to cause nail deformity.[2]

5. Once the biopsy is completed, the proximal nail fold is realigned and sutured back into place.

C. Shave (tangential) biopsy or small excision after nail plate removed

1. Useful to obtain an adequate tissue sample.

2. Avulsion or proximal reflection of nail plate exposes nail matrix and nail bed.

3. Shave (tangential) biopsy matrix.[3,4]

   a. Useful for a broad lesion.

   b. Remove portion of matrix epidermis and dermis. Do not go deep to bone.

   c. Avoids subsequent nail dystrophy, especially if confined to distal matrix only. Distal matrix scar may result in split nail on inferior surface, sometimes seen as longitudinal erythronychia. Split nail (onychoschizia) is due to disruption of

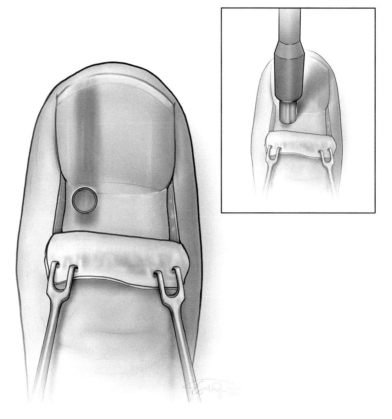

FIGURE 11.9   Single punch technique of distal matrix.

proximal matrix. If biopsy of distal matrix is broad may result in thin nail plate as thickness of nail plate related to matrix vertical dimensions.

    d. Although shallow usually provides adequate tissue for accurate diagnosis.

    e. Place specimen on filter paper before placing in formalin. This keeps specimen flat and helps subsequent orientation for paraffin embedding.[3]

    f. Be mindful that a superficial shave biopsy of a melanoma may not provide complete and accurate Breslow depth and important prognostic data may be lost.[3]

4. Excisional biopsy of matrix (Figure 11.10).

    a. Useful if lesion is small (<5 mm).

    b. Orient longitudinally if possible along length of finger.

    c. Can resuture matrix with 6–0 Vicryl to avoid subsequent nail dystrophy.

5. Shave (tangential) biopsy of nail bed.

    a. Can go to bone but usually unnecessary.

    b. Will not result in nail dystrophy.

6. Excisional biopsy of nail bed (Figure 11.10).

    a. Can do for small or large lesions.

    b. Excisions can be carried to bone.

    c. Try to do fusiform, longitudinally, and laterally if possible to avoid scarring.

    d. Avoid distal matrix if possible.

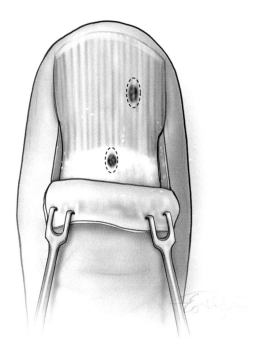

FIGURE 11.10 Orientation of fusiform excisions of nail bed and nail matrix.

  e. If small, may be stitched with polypropylene or nylon suture.

  f. If excision size is large, the wound is difficult to stitch closed. May be allowed to heal by granulation and epidermization.

VIII. Longitudinal Nail Unit Excision

 A. Excision of the nail plate and its adnexa can be complicated and the choice of technique is often determined by the type and location of the lesion.

  1. An atypical pigmented longitudinal lesion adjacent to lateral nail fold.

   a. Can be excised in part (if wide >6 mm) or in total (if narrow <6 mm) with the nail matrix, nail bed, proximal nail fold, and lateral nail fold. The subsequent wound is sutured from the remaining lateral nail fold to nail plate (Figure 11.11).

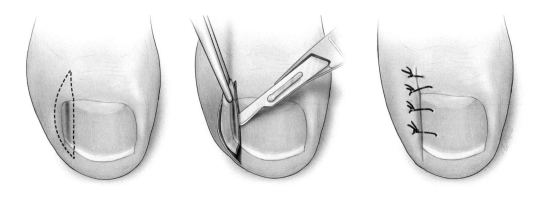

FIGURE 11.11 Excision of lateral nail fold.

       i.   A longitudinal en bloc curvilinear excision that allows for the subsequent histologic examination of the nail plate and its adnexa (proximal nail fold, matrix, bed, and hyponychium) as one unit.

      ii.   It is important to completely excise the lateral matrix ("the horn").[3,4]

    iii.   It is essential to orient on filter paper the nail and its adnexa for the dermatopathologist and to explicitly request that a longitudinal rather than cross section is cut for paraffin embedded sections.[3]

> It is very important to orient a longitudinal nail excision for the dermatopathologist.

     iv.   When healed, the longitudinal excision results in a narrowed nail plate.

  2.   A pigmented streak down the middle of the nail.

     a.   Oftentimes the best approach is to avulse the nail and reflect back the posterior nail fold (Figure 11.6). As the proximal nail fold is reflected proximally, the pigmented streak may be seen to extend into the matrix. At that point an excision is done if indicated; the matrix may be sutured to avoid nail dystrophy.

  3.   An ingrown nail (onychocryptosis).

     a.   Usually results from a nail spicule embedded in lateral nail fold tissue or excess curvature of the nail plate.

     b.   If minimal, may be correctable by insertion of cotton under lateral nail plate.

     c.   If extreme, the proximal nail fold, lateral matrix, lateral nail plate, and lateral nail fold must be removed. If very inflamed or purulent, we recommend antibiotics for a few days prior to and after surgery.

     d.   Note that on removal it is important to remove completely the lateral matrix, sometimes called the "horn". A small curette may be useful to ensure this part of the matrix is removed. If this small portion of matrix remains, it will produce a nail spicule that can be annoying to the patient.[4]

     e.   Results in a narrowed nail plate.

     f.   Bleeding is usually stopped by electrocoagulation.

     g.   The remaining lateral nail fold is stitched to the nail plate. To facilitate passage of the suture needle through the nail plate a small hole can be made by twirling an 11-blade tip through the nail plate.[4]

  4.   Miscellaneous dermatologic diseases of nail unit.

     a.   There are several dermatologic diseases of the nails that are diagnosed or confirmed with a longitudinal excision of the lateral nail fold, nail matrix, nail fold, nail bed, and nail (e.g., psoriasis, lichen planus, etc.).

     b.   This procedure is similar to that for an ingrown nail as above (see VIII.A.3).

     c.   As with pigmented lesions orientation and grossing of the excision specimen is essential to make the right diagnosis.

IX. Postoperative Bleeding

  A. Can usually be controlled by continuously applying pressure for 20 minutes without peeking.

  B. Electrocoagulation may be used but avoid on matrix.

  C. Oxidized regenerated cellulose gauze (Surgicel® Original, Ethicon, Switzerland) or absorbable gelatin sponge (Gelfoam®, Pfizer, Kalamazoo, MI) may be useful.

X. Postoperative Wound Care

  A. Apply an ointment, nonadherent bandage, gauze for pressure, and paper tape.

    1. The surgeon should apply the dressing.

2. We do **not** recommend or use stretchable tubular dressings (e.g., Surgitube® Tubular Gauze [Derma Sciences, Inc., Princeton, NJ], X-Span® Tubular Dressing [Jorgensen Laboratories, Inc., Loveland, CO], Surgilast® Tubular Dressing [Derma Sciences, Inc., Princeton, NJ]) as these may restrict digital blood supply.

> To avoid necrosis, do not use bandages that cause excessive compression on digits after surgery.

3. We do **not** recommend self-adhesive elastic tape dressings (Coban™ [3M, Minneapolis, MN], Hypafix® [BSN Medical, Hamburg, Germany]) as these also might restrict digital blood flow.

4. Tape is cut and applied obliquely and not circumferentially so as not to restrict the blood supply.

5. Dressing is changed daily. At the time of dressing change cleanse with hydrogen peroxide (3%) or normal saline on a cotton tipped applicator. Then apply ointment, a nonadhesive dressing material, paper tape.

6. Patient may get wound wet after 24 hours.

7. Postoperative pain may be considerable especially during first 2 days postoperatively. Therefore, pain medication (narcotic analgesics or nonsteroidal antiinflammatories) may be prescribed. Also, elevation of hand with a sling may decrease pain.[3] Resting hand propped against a pillow on abdomen at night will minimize pain. For feet, an open-toed shoe is helpful.

XI. Common Lesions of the Nail and Nail Apparatus

A. Basal cell carcinoma

1. Very rare.

2. Appears as scaly patch on nail folds similar to Bowen disease carcinoma.

3. Best removed by Mohs micrographic surgery.

B. Digital mucous cyst

1. Due to extrusion of synovium from nearby joint space. Cyst almost never midline because extrusion to either side of extensor tendon.

2. If under proximal nail fold, can cause longitudinal groove in nail plate.

3. Will spontaneously disappear with sudden trauma, e.g., accidentally hitting area on hard surface.

4. Drainage or injection with triamcinolone acetonide (Kenalog®, Bristol-Myers-Squibb, Princeton, NJ) 10 mg/cc can be tried but results are unpredictable.

5. Best result with excision done so that stalk connection between digital mucous cyst and nearby joint synovium is also excised.

a. A bone rongeur can also be used to remove a nearby associated prominent osteophyte but is rarely necessary.

C. Exostosis

1. Appears as distal lateral nail elevation.

2. Confirm with x-ray.

3. Usually on toes, rare on fingers.

4. After removal of distal nail plate, exostosis easily excised by dissection with blunt tipped scissors from underlying bone. A bone rongeur can also be used but is usually unnecessary.

D. Fibrokeratoma

1. Well defined growth underneath proximal nail fold.

2. Usually results in a grooved longitudinal defect in nail plate.

3. Can be easily removed by blunt dissection with blunt tipped scissors. Reflection of the proximal nail fold may be necessary.

E. Glomus tumor

1. Usually painful lesion of nail bed.

2. Appears as small (<5 mm) reddish round lesion under nail plate.

3. Most common tumor of nail bed.

4. Treated by excision after nail plate avulsion.

F. Hemorrhage of nail bed

1. Appears as blue/black area under nail. May see purple streaks in nail plate.

2. Oftentimes mistaken for melanocytic lesion.

3. May appear as pigmented streak in nail plate.

4. If small usually never any pain and patient does not recall injury. Oftentimes injury to toenail bed occurred with new shoes.

> The 11-blade works well to drill a small hole in nail to release a painful hematoma.

5. On biopsy, see collections of erythrocytes, hemosiderin, and plasma under nail plate.

6. If large and acute (during first 24–36 hours) may be quite painful.

    a. Pain removed by trephining through nail plate. We prefer 11-blade taped to wooden end of cotton tipped applicator. As wooden stick is twirled, the blade tip drills through nail gradually until blood release suddenly occurs.

G. Malalignment of the great toenail

1. Nail growth is oriented obliquely and laterally rather than parallel to the direction of underlying bone.

2. Nail plate often has oyster shell conchyliform (conchoidal, conchiform) appearance.

3. May be congenital or acquired from trauma to matrix.

4. Causes pain that is relieved by nail avulsion.

5. Although suggested, matrix realignment is of questionable value.

6. May spontaneously improve after nail avulsion.

H. Melanoma

1. Dark, wide pigmented streak or pigmentation of nail matrix and bed. Has blurred edges. Sometimes triangular in shape.

2. Most commonly found on thumbs or great toe.

3. Melanoma is usually >3–6 mm and often involves pigmentation of proximal or lateral nail fold, which is sometimes referred to as "melanotic whitlow" or "Hutchinson's sign". However, the true Hutchinson's sign is interstitial keratitis associated with congenital syphilis. Another term used is the "pseudo-Hutchinson sign", which refers to brown/black pigment seen through the thin cuticle and eponychium from the nail matrix below.[4] Based on knowledge that Hutchinson's sign is a misnomer, the pseudo-Hutchinson's sign then becomes the pseudopseudo-Hutchinson's sign.

4. Diagnosis made by punch biopsy of matrix either through nail plate or open biopsy after transverse reflection or avulsion of nail plate.

5. For pigmented lesions, look head-on at nail plate at end of nail with dermatoscope. If pigment is in top part of nail plate, biopsy proximal matrix. If pigment is in bottom part of nail plate, biopsy distal matrix.[4]

6. Histologically, melanoma of the nail matrix and bed can be subtle and difficult to properly diagnose.[5]

    a. Usually melanoma of nail matrix requires removal of entire matrix for cure.

  7. Diagnostic pathology likely in matrix.

  8. Consider Mohs Micrographic Surgery for excision.

I. Melanonychia

  1. A thin (<3 mm) pigmented longitudinal streak of the nail bed and matrix extends along the long axis of the nail.

  2. Sometimes called melanonychia striata in longitudinem – a purely description term.

  3. Has sharp margins.

  4. Rectangular in shape.

  5. If occurs in black or brown or Asian patients, most likely benign. If occurs in multiple nails in these patients, even more likely benign and known as "physiologic melonychia". The most common cause of a pigmented nail streak is a melanotic macule.

  6. If darkens and becomes wider, biopsy to rule out melanoma is considered.

  7. Serial photography is recommended if no biopsy is done.

  8. Measure breadth of streak. Melanoma is rare if streak is <6 mm, even more rare if <3 mm.

  9. Often a diagnostic dilemma. Differential diagnosis includes: melanotic macule (the most common cause),[5] nevus (usually junctional), atypical nevus, melanocytic activation (trauma, drug, dermatologic diseases), hemorrhage, Laugier-Hunziker syndrome, Peutz-Jeghers syndrome, onychomycosis.

  10. The melanocytic macule is composed of a slight increase in melanocytes usually only demonstrated by special stains (e.g., Melan-A, Mart-1, and Sox-10).[5]

J. Onychomycosis – nail fungus

  1. Clipping or scraping nail plate.

    a. Examine under microscope with 20% potassium hydroxide (KOH) for hyphae.

    b. Place on Sabouraud dextrose agar. As an alternative, Dermatophyte Test Medium (DTM; Hardy Diagnostics, Santa Maria, CA) is convenient and may be used. This medium contains an antibacterial agent and cycloheximide as well as phenol red as a pH indicator. Since most dermatophytes release alkaline metabolites within a week or two, the medium turns red. However, there can be false positives and false negatives.

    c. Send nail clipping for histopathologic examination with periodic acid Schiff (PAS) stain to rule out fungus.

K. Paronychia

  1. Inflammation involving the proximal and/or lateral nail folds.

  2. Sometimes occurs after manicure or pedicure.

  3. Often associated with infection, usually *Staphylococcus aureus.*

  4. If red and fluctuant, treated by lifting nail fold with an 11-blade and allowing pus to drain. Selective use of appropriate antibiotics is also indicated.

L. Pyogenic granuloma

  1. Usually on lateral nail fold.

  2. Occurs with trauma or associated with pregnancy.

  3. Usually treated by curetting lesion and electrocoagulation of lesion base.

M. Squamous cell carcinoma

  1. Usually appears as scaly patch on lateral and proximal nail folds. Histologically is usually Bowen disease carcinoma.

    2. If Bowen disease carcinoma, associated with human papilloma virus (HPV) 16, 18.

    3. Best removed by Mohs micrographic surgery to preserve nail unit.

N. Verruca

    1. Involves nail folds and often extends into nail bed underneath nail plate.

    2. Treated by liquid nitrogen, which is very painful, or curettage.

    3. If recurrent, nail plate needs to be removed and nail bed as well as nail fold curetted and electrocoagulated. If the wart is large, it may be easier and more efficacious to electrocoagulate the wart first so as to soften and separate it from the surrounding tissue. Then curettage is easier and the curette easily separates and "shells out" the wart.

    4. If multiply recurrent, may consider excision with Mohs micrographic surgery.

Conclusion

The nail unit is complex and requires a specialized knowledge to address problems that arise within it. Some dermatologists have become experts in nail disease – perhaps they could be called onychodermatologists or onychologists.

REFERENCES

1. Scher RK, Daniel CR III. Nails: Therapy, Diagnosis, Surgery. W.B. Saunders Co, Philadelphia, 1990.
2. Jellinek N. Nail Surgery: Practical Tips and Treatment Options. Dermatol Ther 2007; 20: 68–74.
3. Jellinek N. Nail Matrix Biopsy of Longitudinal Melanonychia: Diagnostic Algorithm Including the Matrix Shave Biopsy. J Am Acad Dermatol 2007; 56: 803–810.
4. Jellinek NJ, Velez NF. Dermatologic Manifestations of the Lower Extremity Nail Surgery. Clin Podiatry Med Surg 2016; 33: 319–336.
5. Massi G, LeBoit P. Histopathological Diagnosis of Nevi and Melanoma. Springer, New York, 2014.

Section III

Reconstructive Dermatologic Surgery

12

Skin Grafts

Ken K. Lee

Introduction

Skin grafts are commonly used in skin reconstruction.[1–3] The defining features of a skin graft are its complete detachment from the donor site and the need for new vessel ingrowth into the graft for survival at the recipient site.

I. General Skin Graft Concepts
   A. Skin graft types (Table 12.1)
      1. Full thickness skin graft (FTSG): epidermis plus entire underlying dermis.
      2. Split thickness skin graft (STSG): epidermis plus partial thickness of underlying dermis.
      3. Composite graft: epidermis + dermis + cartilage or other structures.
   B. Definitions
      1. Donor site: the area from which the graft is harvested.
      2. Recipient site: the defect into which the graft is placed and usually sutured.
   C. Advantages
      1. Covers a skin defect with minimal surrounding skin distortion.
      2. Able to cover large defects.
      3. Numerous donor site options.
   D. Disadvantages
      1. Long (4–8 weeks) healing time.
      2. Two areas to heal (donor site and recipient site).
      3. Healed graft may have poor texture and color match to the skin surrounding the recipient site.
II. Stages of Graft Survival
   A. Imbibition – immediate graft absorption of plasma through osmosis from wound bed. Occurs in first 24–48 hours. Bolster improves osmosis.
   B. Inosculation – establishment of anastomoses between graft vessels and endothelial buds in wound bed. Blood flows into graft within about 48–72 hours.
   C. Neovascularization – new capillary ingrowth from wound bed into graft. Occurs in 6–7 days.
   D. Maturation – takes up to 1 year.
III. Full Thickness Skin Graft (FTSG)
   A. Definition
      1. Intact epidermis and entire dermis (Figure 12.1). Thus dermal adnexal structures remain with skin graft.

TABLE 12.1

Comparison between Split Thickness Skin Graft (STSG) and Full Thickness Skin Graft (FTSG)

	STSG	FTSG
Thickness	Thin, epidermis and part of dermis	Thick, epidermis and whole dermis
Survival	Greater, thinner tissue to revascularize	Less, thicker tissue to revascularize
Appearance	Often poor, because it lacks full dermis and skin appendages	Good, but color and texture match to surrounding skin may be variable
Contraction	Common	Unusual
Indications	Large defect or one with limited vascular supply	Small defects with good vascular supply
Recipient Sites	Hands, feet, ears, and over joints	Face especially ears, nose, and lower eyelids
Donor Sites	Medial inner thigh, buttocks, and abdomen	Postauricular sulcus, preauricular sulcus, concha, supraclavicular area, inferior anteriolateral neck, upper eyelid

B. Advantages and indications

  1. Indicated for facial defects where a flap would result in undue morbidity or distortion.

  2. Closer color and texture match to the surrounding recipient site skin than that resulting from a STSG.

  3. Prevents wound contraction if placed within a few days after creating the recipient wound.

  4. Common recipient defect sites include:

    a. Nose.

    b. Rim of the ear.

A full thickness skin graft provides a closer color and texture match to skin surrounding the recipient site than that provided by a split thickness skin graft.

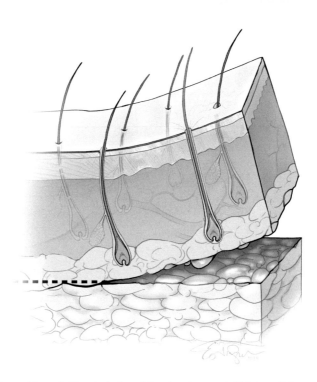

FIGURE 12.1 Full thickness skin graft. Note inclusion of fat when harvested. This fat will be removed before graft is placed into recipient bed.

      c. Lower eyelid.

      d. Large defect on other parts of the face.

      e. Dorsal hand or finger.

  5. Typical donor sites include:

      a. Postauricular sulcus.

      b. Preauricular crease.

      c. Concha of the ear.

      d. Upper eyelid.

      e. Supraclavicular area (for large defects).

      f. Anterolateral neck.

      g. Excised redundant triangular shaped skin ("Burow's triange") that occurs with sliding flap closure.

  6. No special instruments required to harvest graft.

C. Disadvantages and contraindications

  1. Texture and color match to surrounding recipient site skin is variable and unpredictable.

  2. FTSG placement in deep recipient wound may result in a concave skin graft.

  3. Round scar outline of the graft can be noticeable. This scar can be made less apparent by enlarging the recipient defect to include the entire cosmetic unit/subunit or smoothing out the healed graft edge by laser or dermabrasion to blend in with the surrounding normal skin.

  4. Requires a healthy vascular bed. Typically will not survive on bare bone, tendon, or cartilage, all of which are avascular. However, if avascular tissue is a small part of the wound, skin graft will probably survive over this part by "bridging".

  5. Grafts typically take 4–8 weeks to heal completely.

  6. Underlying co-morbidities such as diabetes and smoking may adversely affect graft survival and healing.

D. Technique

  1. To size the graft precisely, a template of the recipient defect is cut from a piece of a non-adherent dressing (e.g., Telfa™ [Covidien, Dublin, Ireland] or suture packet foil).

  2. Template is placed on the donor site skin.

  3. Skin graft is incised around template slightly larger than the template to account for contraction during wound healing. Then the donor skin graft is excised from its bed. Some fat is normally attached to the bottom of the excised skin graft.

  4. Once the skin graft is excised, all fat is trimmed from its bottom (Figure 12.2).

  5. Skin graft is placed into the recipient wound bed and sutured to the surrounding skin. To ensure good contact with the underlying wound, bed tacking sutures through the skin graft to the wound bed are placed as needed.

  6. To ensure the skin graft is kept moist, an antibiotic ointment and nonstick dressing is applied over the graft. The nonstick dressing should extend beyond the suture line.

  7. A tie-over bolster dressing is often placed over the nonstick dressing to provide continuous pressure on the graft so it is immobilized and securely apposed to the underlying wound bed. This bolster dressing is left in place for 1 week and must be kept dry.

  8. The donor site wound is sutured with dermal/subdermal sutures and dermal/epidermal stitches.

IV. Split Thickness Skin Graft (STSG)

  A. Definition

    1. Intact epidermis and partial dermis.

      a. Varying thicknesses defined by thousandths of an inch (Figure 12.3).

        i. Thin – 0.008–0.012 inch (0.2 mm–0.3 mm).

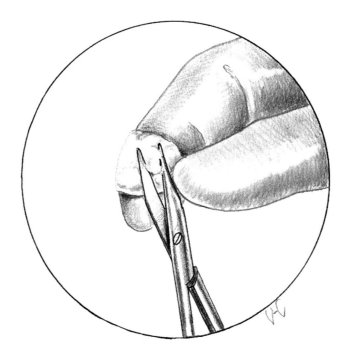

FIGURE 12.2 Fat trimmed from full thickness skin graft using tenotomy scissors.

      ii.   Medium – 0.012–0.018 inch (0.3 mm–0.5 mm).

      iii. Thick – 0.018–0.030 inch (0.5 mm–0.8 mm).

   d. Selection of STSG thickness varies with likelihood of vascularization (thin STSG preferred if likelihood is less) and amount of cushioning needed (e.g., on bottom of foot a thick STSG would increase cushioning effect).

B. Advantages and indications

   1. Indicated for large wound defects where a full thickness skin graft or flap is not feasible or practical.

   2. Often more functional than skin flap reconstruction.

   3. Vascularizes faster than a full thickness skin graft.

   4. Can be fenestrated or meshed to increase the STSG size.

   5. Increased likelihood of survival compared to that of a full thickness skin graft.

   6. Because it is thin, a STSG can be placed to monitor a wound for recurrence of an aggressive skin cancer. A flap, a FTSG, or granulation can "bury" an underlying skin cancer thereby increasing the time until it is noticed.

> A split thickness skin graft provides a "window" to monitor an underlying wound for tumor recurrence.

   7. Typical recipient wound sites:

      a. Any large wound area that has a vascular bed.

   8. Typical donor sites – areas covered by clothing.

      a. Upper inner thigh.

      b. Buttock.

      c. Abdomen.

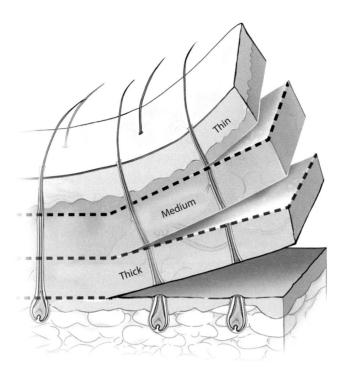

FIGURE 12.3 Various thicknesses of split thickness skin grafts.

C. Disadvantages and contraindications
  1. Usually requires specialized instruments to harvest graft.
  2. Poor color and texture match to the skin surrounding recipient site compared to a full thickness skin graft because a STSG lacks complete dermis and skin appendages. After healing, typically appears hypopigmented, atrophic, and indented.
  3. STSG is fragile and the underlying wound needs to be immobilized (important over joints).
     a. Requires healthy vascular bed. Typically will not survive on bare bone, tendon, or cartilage.
     b. STSG typically takes 4–8 weeks to heal completely.
     c. May result in recipient wound contraction, especially if not placed immediately after recipient wound created.
     d. Underlying co-morbidities such as diabetes, smoking, and poor diet (especially in elderly) may impact survival of a STSG and healing of its donor site.
     e. The donor site wound is superficial and left open to heal by granulation and epidermization using dressings. Donor site wound healing often is more of a problem in terms of pain and dressings than the STSG at the recipient site.
D. Technique
  1. Recipient site is sized either by measuring directly or by means of a template made from a piece of non-adherent dressing (e.g., Telfa™).
  2. The donor site is marked to the size of the recipient site by using a ruler or the prior cut template. In order to compensate for contraction, the graft should be approximately 25% larger than the template unless the graft is meshed or heavily fenestrated.

3. Harvesting techniques.

    a. Free hand with a 10 scalpel blade. Limited to harvesting small grafts and can result in uneven graft thicknesses.

    b. Free hand with a Weck knife or a Silver dermatome. Useful for small to medium size grafts. Can vary the graft thickness by using different size guides or adjustment screws.

    c. Electric dermatomes – e.g.: Zimmer, Padgett, Brown dermatomes. Indicated for larger skin grafts. Can precisely adjust dermatome to cut graft at uniform thickness.

    d. Mesher – for very large defects, meshing the graft allows for significant expansion of the graft for greater wound coverage.

4. To ensure an easy glide of the dermatome, the skin is thinly lubricated with a sterile ointment, such as Polysporin®.

5. When harvesting, continuous traction is placed on the skin surrounding the donor site to ensure uniform graft thickness (Figure 12.4).

6. A STSG is sutured to the skin surrounding the wound. To ensure adequate contact with the underlying bed, several tacking sutures are placed through the STSG to the wound bed.

7. To prevent dead space underneath the graft at the wound periphery, stitch the graft so that it completely abuts the recipient wound edge. This is important because the recipient wound is typically deeper than the graft thickness. A good stitch for this purpose is the vertical or horizontal mattress stitch.

8. Small incisions are often made in the STSG to allow drainage and prevent fluid or blood accumulation underneath the graft.

9. To ensure the STSG is kept moist, an antibiotic ointment and nonstick dressing is applied over the STSG. This dressing typically extends beyond the graft wound edge by a centimeter.

10. A tie-over bolster dressing is placed over the nonstick dressing. This bolster dressing is left in place for 1 week.

V. Composite Skin Grafts

  A. Definition

    1. Skin and cartilage.

    2. Usually harvested from anterior helix or antihelix. From these locations usually includes skin on both sides of cartilage.

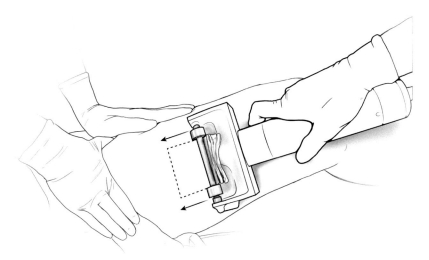

FIGURE 12.4 Harvesting split thickness skin graft with Padgett dermatome. Note traction being applied by assistant to flatten surrounding skin.

B. Advantages
1. Excellent color and texture match for small (<1 cm) through-and-through defects in nasal ala.
2. Restores missing skin, cartilage or fibrocartilage, and mucosa, and maintains tissue architecture. Thus adds bulk and structural support.

C. Disadvantages
1. High likelihood of graft failure due to avascular tissue (cartilage) and a small recipient graft bed.
2. Graft size is limited to 2 cm or less to decrease necrosis risk.

D. Technique
1. Graft harvested from anterior helix or antihelix same size as full thickness ala defect.
2. Donor site allowed to heal or reconstructed with a skin flap.
3. Posterior (inside) graft sutured first to mucosa.
4. Pockets made on either side of recipient wound where graft cartilage is inserted and sutured to alar cartilage with absorbable suture.
5. Outside part of graft sutured to skin and mucosa.
6. Continuous application of ice pack for the first 24 hours may decrease the metabolic demands on the composite graft and increase the probability of survival.

VI. Problems and Complications with Skin Grafts

A. Immediate problems/complications
1. Full thickness necrosis:
   a. All or part of the graft does not vascularize and remains white.
   b. Best results if necrotic graft is kept in place and moist until wound completely heals. To keep the necrotic graft moist an ointment and dressing is applied daily until healing is complete.

   If a skin graft becomes necrotic, best results are obtained by keeping it moist and covered on all sides with daily dressing changes until the underlying wound heals completely.

2. Partial necrosis.
   a. Epidermal blistering indicates superficial necrosis only. Graft will probably survive.
   b. Best results if graft is kept moist with daily dressings until graft completely heals.

B. Delayed problems/complications
1. Erythema and telangiectasias – usually resolves in 3–6 months. Can be treated with a vascular laser; that is, a laser that targets vascular tissue.
2. Hypertrophic wound edges – resolves with time (6 months to 1 year) or may be treated with triamcinolone acetonide (Kenalog-10®) injection for faster resolution and/or pressure massage.
3. Irregular wound edges – may be removed with dermabrasion or an ablative CO_2 laser.
4. Whole graft hypertrophic – if it does not respond to time and triamcinolone acetonide injection (Kenalog-10®), may require revisional surgery, such as excision of excess scar tissue underlying the graft.

Conclusion

Skin grafts are an important part of the reconstructive armamentarium used in dermatologic surgery. One must understand their advantages and disadvantages in order to best utilize them to their fullest capacity. Proper technique is paramount to ensure skin graft survival and to achieve the best cosmetic and functional outcome.

REFERENCES

1. Glogau RG, Haas AF. Skin graft. In: Local Flaps in Facial Reconstruction (Baker SR, Swanson NA, editors). Mosby, Inc, St. Louis, 1995; 247–271.
2. Lee KK, Swanson NA, Lee HN. Overview of grafts. In: Color Atlas of Cutaneous Excisions and Repairs. Cambridge University Press, New York, 2008; 51–58.
3. Skouge JW. Skin Grafting. Churchill-Livingstone, New York, 1991.

13

Cutaneous Flaps

Jonathan L. Cook

Introduction

Flaps are movable constructs of skin and subcutaneous tissue with an attached blood supply used to repair skin and soft tissue wounds. In dermatologic surgery, most flaps are used to reconstruct deep, complex wounds that result from extirpation of skin cancers. The main advantage of skin flap repairs is their ability to shift tissue from a nearby area where skin is loose and transfer it into an area where skin is tight. Unlike skin grafts, skin flaps are harvested from tissue near or immediately adjacent to the operative wound and provide an excellent texture and color match to the skin around the defect to be repaired. Flaps also retain some amount of predictable perfusion by incorporating deeper vascular structures within their bases. This predictable perfusion allows complicated flaps to be used and the resultant excellent texture and color match offer surgeons and patients aesthetic results typically far superior to the aesthetic results seen with simple wound management strategies.

I. Some of the Various Historical Classification Schemata for Flaps – all classification schemata have significant limitations.
- A. By vascular supply
  1. Random pattern flaps (Figure 13.1A): flaps relying on the highly anastomotic subdermal vascular plexus for perfusion – the majority of flaps used in dermatologic surgery.[1]
  2. Axial pattern flaps (Figure 13.1B): flaps with a large, named artery in their bases.
  3. Myocutaneous flaps (Figure 13.1C): flaps utilizing a muscle that provides additional vascular supply.
  4. Fasciocutaneous flaps (Figure 13.1D): flaps utilizing arteries and veins originating in underlying muscles; these vessels perforate muscle fascia and supply the overlying skin flap.
- B. By primary motion
  1. Advancement (Figure 13.2A).
  2. Rotation (Figure 13.2B).
  3. Transposition (Figure 13.2C).
  4. Interpolation.

    There are many useful ways to categorize skin flaps.
- C. By flap shape/configuration
  1. Bilobed flap.
     - a. 45° (Figure 13.3A).
     - b. 90° (Figure 13.3B).
  2. Rhombic/rhomboid flap (Figure 13.2C).
  3. Banner flap.
  4. Hatchet flap.

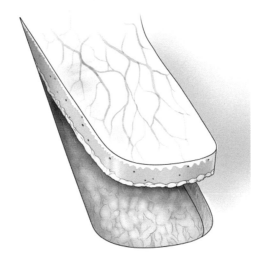

Random pattern skin flap

FIGURE 13.1A   Random pattern skin flap. Vascularization does not depend on any one artery.

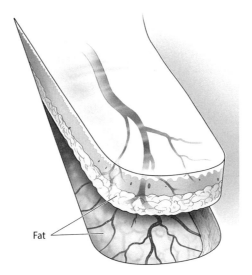

Fat

Axial pattern skin flap

FIGURE 13.1B   Axial pattern skin flap. Vascularization depends on one artery.

    D. By eponymous designation
        1. Abbé flap.
        2. Mustardé flap.
        3. Rieger flap.
        4. Tenzel flap.
        5. Tripier flap.

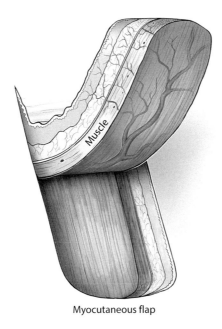

Myocutaneous flap

FIGURE 13.1C Myocutaneous flap. Vascularization derived from arteries from muscle underlying skin.

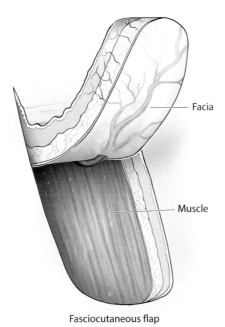

Fasciocutaneous flap

FIGURE 13.1D Fasciocutaneous flap. Vascularization derived from arteries in underlying muscle fascia.

    E. By donor site
        1. Forehead flap.
            a. Median (Figure 13.4A).
            b. Paramedian (Figure 13.4B).
        2. Cheek transposition flap.

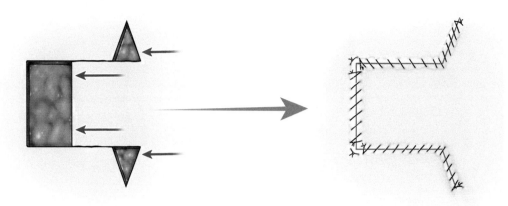

FIGURE 13.2A   Advancement flap. Direction of flap is parallel to the maximum skin tension lines.

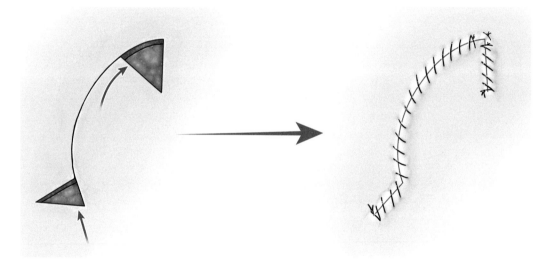

FIGURE 13.2B   Rotational flap. Direction of flap is parallel to the maximum skin tension lines.

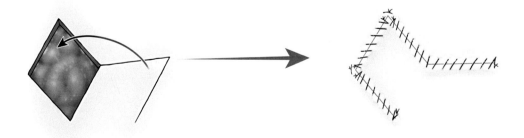

FIGURE 13.2C   Rhombic transposition flap. Direction of flap is perpendicular to the maximum skin tension lines.

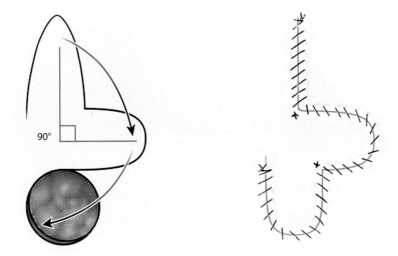

FIGURE 13.3A   90° bilobed flap. This flap produces excess tissue bunching (dog ear) at the flap base.

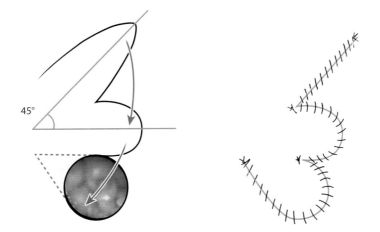

FIGURE 13.3B   45° bilobed flap. This flap has less tissue bunching than the 90° bilobed flap at the flap base.

    F. By location
        1. Local.
        2. Regional.
        3. Distant.
    Regardless of the flap classification scheme used, there are various definitions and concepts common to all flap repairs (Table 13.1).

  II. The Physiologic Basis for Flap Survival/Success:
    A. The baseline vascular perfusion of skin supplies up to 10x its basic metabolic needs.
        1. This perfusion redundancy allows the severing of much of the skin blood supply without producing tissue death.
    B. Skin perfusion is largely dependent on a rich, highly anastomotic subdermal plexus of vessels.

Sufficient blood supply is critical to skin flap survival.

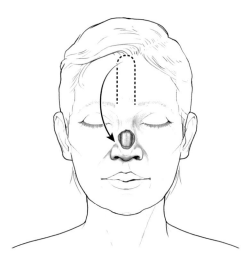

FIGURE 13.4A Median forehead flap. This flap results in an imperceptible scar in the forehead.

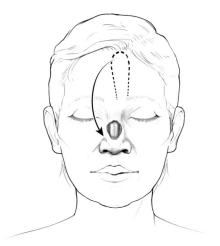

FIGURE 13.4B Paramedian forehead flap. This flap has less rotational torsion than the median forehead flap.

    C. Sufficient perforating vessels, sometimes through muscles, must be preserved within an elevated flap base to ensure flap survival.

    D. Perfusion predictably falls directly along the length of a flap as the distance increases from the high perfusion pressure vessels in the flap base.

    E. Wound closure tension and flap perfusion are inversely correlated.[2,3]

  III. Advantages of Flap Repairs

    A. Flaps often produce superior aesthetic and functional results.

    B. Because a flap has an intact blood supply, it has a high likelihood of survival.

    C. Deep wounds are able to be repaired with thick flaps.

    D. Flaps can prevent distortion and can be used to cover relatively avascular tissue such as bone or cartilage.

  IV. Disadvantages of Flap Repairs

    A. Require additional nearby incision lines.

    B. May not survive despite proper design and execution.

TABLE 13.1

Skin Flap Terminology

Primary Defect	Surgical wound to be repaired; the recipient site
Secondary Defect	Surgical wound created when skin flap is cut and moved; flap donor site
Primary Lobe	Portion of flap that covers primary defect
Secondary Lobe	Additional lobe that covers secondary defect
Pivot Point	Point at flap base around which the flap rotates
Tip	Triangular piece of tissue at flap's leading edge
Base	Proximal area of flap that is not incised; usually contains blood supply to flap
Tension Vector	Direction of force when moving primary flap lobe into primary defect
Primary Motion	Main directional movement of flap, e.g., advancement, rotation
Secondary Motion	Directional movement different from primary motion
Key Stitch	Stitch that initially positions and takes tension off flap
Anchoring Stitch	A stitch that goes from flap to underlying tissue so that flap becomes contoured to underlying concavity or positions flap to take tension off the recipient site. Also known as a pexing or tacking suture
Dog Ear	Soft tissue protrusion due to tissue buckling when flap moves; sometimes called standing or lying cone

    C.   May cause disfigurement or function problems if improperly designed.

    D.   Require extensive undermining which introduces the risk of surgical trauma and intra- and post-operative hemorrhage.

    E.   May need a revision or a second stage repair.

    F.   Flaps can be expensive.

  V. Basic Design Suggestions for Most Facial Flaps

    A.   No wound should ever be reconstructed with a flap repair until confirmation of tumor-free margins has been obtained (ideally with Mohs micrographic surgery – see Chapter 14).

    B.   Always select the simplest reconstructive alternative – never use a flap if the wound would heal well with second intention or with a simple linear repair.

    C.   Determine every patient's aesthetic expectations and willingness to undergo a more complicated reconstructive procedure.

    D.   Select patients and operative sites carefully – flap ischemia can be much more frequent in heavy smokers, in patients with severe vascular disease and general debility, and in scarred or previously irradiated tissue. Also, areas with less vascular supply, such as the lower legs, are more likely to necrose.

    E.   Identify all areas of available tissue excess near the surgical wound that could serve as suitable flap donor sites.

  VI. Basic Execution Suggestions for Most Facial Flaps

    A.   Sharply incise the flap along its previously demarcated design to the depth of the deep subcutaneous fat.

    B.   Widely undermine the flap to improve flap motion and to minimize tension on the distal, ischemically prone portion of the flap.[4]

    C.   Achieve meticulous and complete hemostasis prior to closing the flap and its donor site.

    D.   Place an initial buried suture either at the point of maximal flap tension near its insertion point or at the flap donor site.

    E.   Do not trim any excess skin until the flap has been accurately and completely inset.

    F. Handle all tissue, particularly the epidermal edges, infrequently and delicately, using atraumatic surgical instruments.

    G. Place several buried dermal/subdermal sutures to take tension off of and to precisely approximate the epidermal wound edges.

    H. Close the epidermal edges of the flap with non-absorbable or absorbable cutaneous sutures.

    I. Instruct the patient in the importance of proper wound care, which can have dramatic influence on flap success.

Gentle tissue handling is essential to successful skin flaps.

VII. A Few Typical Flaps

    A. Advancement flap (Figure 13.2A)

      1. A simple rectangular flap that utilizes unidirectional advancement. Often used in the eyebrow or on the forehead.

    B. Rotation flap (Figure 13.2B)

      1. A curvilinear flap used to rotate adjacent tissue laxity into an operative wound. Often used on the cheek and scalp.

    C. Rhombic transposition flap (Figure 13.2C)

      1. A geometric flap to one side of a rhombic-shaped defect often used in the central face, including the nose, medial and lateral canthus, and cheek.

    D. Bilobed transposition flap (Figures 13.3A and B)

      1. A geometrically complicated dual lobe transposition flap used most commonly on the rounded nosetip.[5] The 90° bilobed flap (Figure 13.3A) is rarely used. The 45° bilobed flap (Figure 13.3B) is the preferred design.

    E. Forehead flap (Figures 13.4A and B)

      1. An axially patterned flap with the supratrochlear artery as its vascular supply at the flap pivot point near the medial brow. Used for the reconstruction of large deep distal nasal wounds in which there is insufficient adjacent tissue laxity to allow for a local repair. The median forehead flap (Figure 13.4A) is preferred by some surgeons as it results in a cosmetically superior forehead donor site scar. The paramedian forehead flap (Figure 13.4B) has become popular because it can be used on patients with a small forehead and results in less kinking when the flap is transposed to the recipient site.

Conclusion

Flaps offer dermatologic surgeons unparalleled opportunities to repair both small and large complicated skin cancer excision wounds with predictable success. Proper training and experience are essential to achieve the optimal cosmetic and functional outcome.

REFERENCES

1. Cook JL, Goldman GD. Random pattern cutaneous flaps. In: Surgery of the Skin (Robinson JK et al., editors). Elsevier Mosby, Philadelphia, 2005; 311–344.
2. Dzubow LM. The Dynamics of Flap Movement: The Effect of Pivotal Restraint on Flap Rotation and Transposition. J Dermatol Surg Oncol 1987; 13: 1348–1353.
3. Larrabee WF Jr, Holloway GA Jr, Sutton D. Wound Tension and Blood Flow in Skin Flaps. Ann Otol Rhinol Laryngol 1984; 93: 112–115.
4. Boyer JD, Zitelli JA, Brodland DG. Undermining in Cutaneous Surgery. Dermatol Surg 2001; 27: 75–78.
5. Cook JL. A Review of the Bilobed Flap's Design with Particular Emphasis on the Minimization of Alar Displacement. Dermatol Surg 2000; 26: 354–362.

14

Mohs Micrographic Surgery

Manish Gharia and Brittany Ahuja

Introduction

Mohs micrographic surgery (MMS) is a procedure that allows for microscopically guided tissue resection of skin cancers. MMS has been shown to have the highest cure rates for selected tumors; the technique allows a surgeon to spare as much healthy tissue as possible by excising the cancer in layers until all margins (superficial and deep) are tumor free.

I. History

While working as a research assistant in the 1930s to Professor Michael F. Guyer at the University of Wisconsin, Dr. Frederic Mohs began experimenting with different compounds to determine their curative potential for neoplasms.[1] During his experiments, Dr. Mohs observed that a specially compounded zinc chloride ($ZnCl_2$) paste was able to fix tissue *in vivo* and cause necrosis. After the neoplasm was fixed with $ZnCl_2$ paste, the fixed tissue was excised without pain or bleeding. The excised zinc chloride infused tissue was mapped to correspond to the orientation and location from where it was removed. It was then subdivided into smaller pieces and each piece was cut with a microtome, stained, and viewed under the microscope. The exact tumor location could then be indicated on a drawn map of the excised tissue which corresponded to the same location on the patient. Dr. Mohs named this process of applying zinc chloride paste to a neoplasm, excising it, and microscopically mapping it as "chemosurgery" and treated his first patient on June 23, 1936. The technique chemosurgery has undergone many name changes over the years (Figure 14.1). Today it is commonly referred to as Mohs micrographic surgery, although the Accreditation Council for Graduate Medical Education (ACGME) prefers to eliminate Dr. Mohs' name and simply refers to the technique as micrographic surgery. Nevertheless, the term "Mohs surgery" has persisted and is commonly used today by the majority of physicians.

Although initially Mohs micrographic surgery resulted in high cure rates, a few problems developed. Because of the zinc chloride tissue penetration, pain and inflammation occurred at the surgical site and only one excision and one microscopic examination could be done each day. Furthermore, after the final negative layer the post-operative reconstruction was delayed or not done at all due to the presence of fixed necrotic tissue that took a week or two to separate. Addressing these problems led to the development of the fresh tissue technique, which included the injection of a local anesthetic around the neoplasm prior to excision. The fresh tissue technique was initially named Mohs chemosurgery and solved the problems associated with the fixed tissue technique. The advantages of utilizing this new technique resulted in the elimination of zinc chloride paste and allowed for excision and microscopic examination of multiple tissue layers on the same day if needed.

In 1967, Dr. Mohs founded the American College of Chemosurgery, which was later renamed in 1986 as the American College of Mohs Micrographic Surgery and Cutaneous Oncology. In 1982, the College began oversight of a formalized 1-year fellowship-training program in MMS. MMS is currently the gold standard for skin cancer treatment and offers high cure rates,

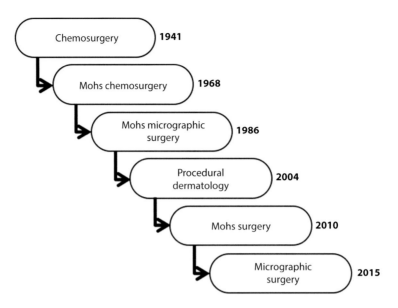

FIGURE 14.1 Evolution of the name micrographic surgery.

while sparing healthy tissue. In 2004, the ACGME took over oversight of the Mohs College fellowship-training programs.

II. Indications for Mohs Micrographic Surgery (Figure 14.2)

In 2012, the American Academy of Dermatology, in cooperation with the American Society for Dermatologic Surgery, extensively studied and published under what circumstances MMS was appropriate.[2] Subsequent consensus studies for basal cell carcinoma and squamous cell carcinoma have been published by the American Society for Dermatologic Surgery.[3,4] Following are the generally agreed upon indications for MMS (Figure 14.2):

A. Incomplete prior treatment

    1. Tumor recurrence after presumptively adequate treatment.

    2. Persistent tumor after inadequate prior treatment.

    3. Incompletely excised tumor on routine pathologic examination ("positive margins").

> The most important indication for Mohs micrographic surgery is tumor recurrence.

B. Aggressive pathology

    1. Poorly differentiated squamous cell carcinoma (SCC).

    2. Deep (>4 mm) SCC.

    3. Infiltrative and morphea-like basal cell carcinoma (BCC).

    4. Melanoma.

    5. Perineural or lymphovascular invasion.

    6. Rare skin tumors (e.g., dermatofibrosarcoma protuberans [DFSP], Merkel cell carcinoma, microcystic adnexal carcinoma, atypical fibroxanthoma/ pleomorphic sarcoma [AFX/PS], extramammary Paget disease [EMPD], sebaceous carcinoma).

C. High reoccurrence risk location

    1. Nonmelanoma skin cancers (NMSCs) located in the "H" zone.[5]

    "H" zone includes the nose, cheek, ears, forehead, perioral, and periocular areas.

    2. Tumors located in areas that are important for functionality (e.g., penis, digits).

    3. Cosmetically important areas where sparing healthy tissue is essential.

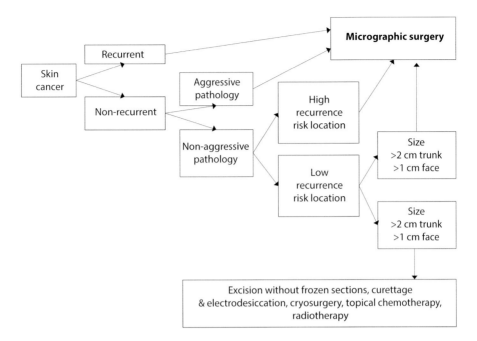

FIGURE 14.2 Skin cancer treatment algorithm for appropriate use of Mohs micrographic surgery.

D. Size
   1. Greater than 2 cm on the trunk.
   2. Greater than 1 cm on the face.
E. Special tumor features
   1. Occurrence within chronic ulcers.
   2. Occurrence within old burns, traumatic scars, chronic ulcers (Marjolin ulcer).
   3. Occurrence within an area of prior radiation.
F. Special patient features
   1. Patients with multiple skin cancers.
   2. Young patients with skin cancer.
   3. Immunocompromised (HIV, transplant) patients.
   4. Patients with genetic syndromes predisposing to skin cancers (e.g., basal cell nevus syndrome, Bloom syndrome, xeroderma pigmentosum).
   5. Tumors within chronic dermatologic conditions (e.g., lichen sclerosus et atrophicus, discoid lupus erythematosus).
   6. Patients with psoriasis treated previously by phototherapy.
III. Steps for Mohs Micrographic Surgery (MMS) (Figure 14.3)
   A. Surgical (Step 1)
      1. Tumor is debulked with a dermal curette to determine subclinical extension of tumor, both peripherally and in depth.
      2. A thin skin layer (about 2 mm) is excised around the debulked area on the skin surface and below the debulked cavity. During this excision the scalpel is angled at about 45° to the skin surface.
         a. 45° angle will allow the peripheral skin margin on the excised tissue to be flattened prior to freezing and cutting microscopic sections in the cryostat.
      3. Bleeding is stopped and a dressing is applied.

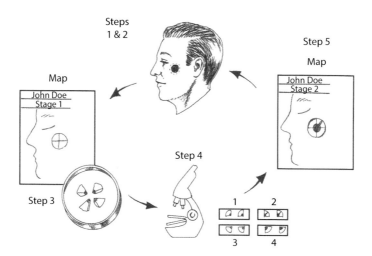

FIGURE 14.3   Steps for Mohs micrographic surgery to remove skin cancer.

B. Mapping (Step 2)
1. A "Mohs" map is drawn that shows the size, location, and orientation of the excised tissue on the patient.
C. Preparation of histologic slides (Step 3)
1. The excised tissue is usually cut vertically into two or more pieces. Each of the subdivided pieces is referred to as a tissue block. Each tissue block is numbered and its number is indicated on the Mohs map.
2. At least two different colored dyes that intersect are applied to the non-epidermal tissue edges.
3. The color of each dye is indicated on the corresponding drawn tissue edges on the Mohs map.
4. Each tissue block is manually flattened on a glass slide with the cut surgical margin including the epidermal edge (if present) directly on the glass slide. The block is frozen to the glass slide using liquid nitrogen.
    a. Flattening the specimen allows for 100% examination of the cut surgical margins, including the epidermis.
5. The glass slide with the stuck on flattened frozen tissue is then inverted and placed on an object disk holder (also known as a "chuck") where the tissue block is released and covered using a tissue medium to hold the specimen on the object disk holder while it is being frozen further in the cryostat.

Unlike routine frozen sections performed in the operating room, Mohs micrographic frozen sections are oriented and cut so that complete epidermis, dermis, and fat are present on each section.

6. Once the tissue block is adequately frozen, the microtome in the cryostat is used to cut thin (5–10 micrometer [μm]) tissue slices (sections) from the frozen tissue block. Care is taken to ensure that if present, the epidermis, dermis, and fat is complete on each section. Generally, 3–6 cut tissue sections are placed on each slide.
7. Slices (sections) are carefully mounted onto a glass slide.
8. The cut tissue slices (sections) on the glass slide are then stained.

      a.   Hematoxylin and eosin (H&E).

         i.   Used to stain squamous cell carcinomas.

        ii.   Eosin highlights keratin found within atypical squamous cells.

      b.   Toluidine Blue (T. Blue).[6]

         i.   Used to stain basal cell carcinomas.

        ii.   Highlights acid mucopolysaccharides and hyaluronic acid which metachromatically appear as a magenta halo around BCC cell nests.

      c.   Oil Red O.[7]

         i.   Used to stain sebaceous gland carcinomas.

      d.   PAS.

         i.   Used to stain extramammary Paget's cells.

      e.   Immunostains.

         i.   MART-1 (melanoma antigen recognized by T-cells). Used to highlight melanosome containing cells which can be melanoma cells.

        ii.   CK-7 for extramammary Paget's cells.

D. Microscopic examination (Step 4–5)

   1. Slides with the stained tissue sections are coverslipped and examined under the microscope (Step 4).

      a.   Any tumor present at the cut surgical margins is identified and marked on the Mohs map corresponding to the exact area where tumor is present on the tissue section (Step 5).

      b.   If tumor is not present on all the tissue sections, the Mohs micrographic surgical procedure is completed.

      c.   If tumor is present, an additional piece or pieces of tissue will be taken from the corresponding area on the patients' wound and the process (Steps 2–5) is repeated.

IV. Wound Repair

  A. First intention: wound is immediately repaired.

   1. Side-to-side closure, either an intermediate or complex repair.

   2. Skin flap.

   3. Skin graft.

  B. Second intention: wound is allowed to heal by itself (see Figure 14.2)

   1. Three phases.

      a.   Granulation.

      b.   Contraction.

      c.   Epidermization.

   2. Used when results will be acceptable and distortion is minimal.

   3. Requires daily dressing changes with ointment and bandage.

   4. Usually takes 6 weeks.

> Select wounds created by Mohs micrographic surgery are sometimes allowed to heal by second intention and often result in an excellent cosmetic outcome.

  C. Third intention: wound repair is delayed and performed before wound is completely healed.

   1. Delay allows wound to fills up with granulation tissue so that wound will not be concave. However, granulation tissue contraction can occur during the delay causing distortion of a free edge such as the nasal alar rim.

   2. Repair with third intention usually performed with a skin graft.

    V. Skin Cancer Types Best Treated with MMS

      A. Basal cell carcinoma

      B. Squamous cell carcinoma

      C. Bowen disease carcinoma

      D. Sebaceous cell carcinoma

      E. Atypical fibroxanthoma/pleomorphic sarcoma

      F. Dermatofibrosarcoma protuberans

      G. Merkel cell carcinoma

      H. Extramammary Paget disease

       I. In-situ melanoma

> Physicians who excise skin cancer and then have the pathologist create and interpret frozen sections are not doing Mohs micrographic surgery.

  VI. Real or Fake Mohs Micrographic Surgery (MMS)

      A. MMS requires that the physician act in two integrated but separate and distinct capacities: surgeon and pathologist.[8] The physician excises the tissue; ensures that the tissue is properly grossed and color-coded; oversees the laboratory to ensure that frozen sections are properly oriented, cut, and stained; and accurately interprets the stained frozen sections and marks tumor on the map. This is real MMS that assesses 100% of the cut surgical margin.

      B. If either of these services is performed by another physician, or healthcare professional, MMS was not done and cannot be billed for.

      C. Physicians sometimes advertise and portray to patients that they perform MMS because frozen sections are performed by a pathologist at the time of surgery. The high cure rates with MMS can only be achieved when 100% of the surgical margin is examined which will not happen when a pathologist routinely processes frozen sections. Furthermore, the surgeon does not examine the frozen sections. Thus, this is fake MMS.

      D. Another common scenario is where a surgeon removes tissue and sends it for permanent sections. If the surgeon draws the map, color codes the sections, places the sections in the cassettes, and interprets the permanent microscopic sections this is considered to be real MMS. Because it takes at least 24 hours to produce permanent sections, this procedure has been labeled "Slow Mohs".

      E. If the surgeon removes tissue and sends it for permanent sections, without orientation and does not function as the pathologist, MMS has not been performed. This is fake MMS.

  VII. Becoming a Mohs Micrographic Surgeon – requires the following:

      A. Medical school (4 years)

      B. Internship (1 year)

      C. Dermatology residency (3 years)

      D. Micrographic surgery and dermatologic oncology fellowship (1 year)

Conclusion

Mohs micrographic surgery is the optimal treatment for a skin cancer that is difficult to cure and that occurs in an area where one wants to preserve as much normal tissue as possible. This technique allows for complete examination of all cut surgical margins and thus results in the highest possible tumor cure rate. Proper training in this technique provides advanced surgical expertise, a comprehensive understanding of oncologic dermatopathology, the ability to create properly oriented and stained frozen sections, and experience with complicated reconstructive procedure.

REFERENCES

1. Trost LB, Bailin PL. History of Mohs Surgery. Dermatol Clin 2011; 29: 135–139.
2. Connolly SM, Baker DR, Coldiron BM et al. Appropriate Use Criteria for Mohs Micrographic Surgery: A Report of the American Academy of Dermatology, American College of Mohs Surgery, American Society for Dermatologic Surgery Association, and the American Society for Mohs Surgery. Dermatol Surg 2012 Oct; 38(10): 1582–1603.
3. Kauvar AN, Cronin T Jr, Roenigk R et al. Consensus for Nonmelanoma Skin Cancer Treatment: Basal Cell Carcinoma, Including a Cost Analysis of Treatment Methods. Dermatol Surg 2015; 41(5): 550–571.
4. Kauvar ANB, Christopher J et al. Consensus for Nonmelanoma Skin Cancer Treatment, Part II: Squamous Cell Carcinoma, Including a Cost Analysis of Treatment Methods. Dermatol Surg 2015; 41(11): 1214–1240.
5. Swanson NA. Mohs Surgery: Technique, Indications, Applications, and the Future. Arch Dermatol 1983; 119: 761–773.
6. Humphreys TR, Nemeth A, McCrevey S et al. A Pilot Study Comparing Toluidine Blue and Hematoxylin and Eosin Staining of Basal Cell and Squamous Cell Carcinoma During Mohs Surgery. Dermatol Surg 1996; 22: 693–697.
7. Miller CJ, Sobanko JF, Zhu X, Nunnciato T, Urban CR. Special Stains in Mohs Surgery. Dermatol Clin 2011; 29(2): 273–286.
8. American Medical Association. CPT: Current Procedural Terminology. American Medical Association, Chicago, IL, 2016; p. 92.

Section IV

Cosmetic Dermatologic Surgery

15

Neurotoxins

Alastair Carruthers and Jean Carruthers

Introduction

Botulinum neurotoxin, the causative agent for botulism, is the most lethal biologic substance known and derives from the gram-negative anaerobic bacterium *Clostridium botulinum*. In the last few decades, the most potent serotypes – types A and B – have been extensively studied and developed for a range of therapeutic and cosmetic indications stemming from the neurotoxin's ability to produce temporary paralysis when injected into muscles.

    I. Pharmacology of Botulinum Neurotoxins[1]

      A. Derived from the bacterium *C. botulinum*

      B. Seven distinct serotypes: A, B, C_1, D, E, F, and G

        1. 150-kD dichain polypeptides; heavy and light chains linked by disulfide bonds.

        2. Each differs with regard to cellular mechanism of action and clinical profile.

        3. Type A has longest duration of neuromuscular paralysis.

      C. Commercially available for medical use: serotype A (Botox, Dysport, Xeomin) and serotype B (Myobloc)

      D. Mechanisms of action

        1. Heavy chain binds toxin to presynaptic receptor sites on motor nerve terminals and helps the neurotoxin cross cell membrane directly or by pinocytosis.

          a. Light chain of serotype A cleaves proteolytically a 25-kD synaptosomal-associated protein (SNAP-25). SNAP-25 is a type of SNARE (synaptosomal-associated protein receptor) proteins. SNARE proteins are involved in exocytosis of acetylcholine. Thus, the light chains interfere with release of acetycholine from presynaptic motor neurons.

          b. Light chain of type B cleaves vesicle-associated membrane protein (VAMP or synaptobrevin).

        2. Inhibits the release from presynaptic motor neurons of acetylcholine and other neurotransmitters, including substance-P, glutamate, and calcitonin gene-related peptide.

   II. Clinical Effects

      A. Flaccid paralysis of the injected musculature. Flaccid paralysis implies loss of muscle tone and absence of tendon reflexes

      B. Area of denervation about 2.5 cm around point of injection

      C. Effects appear within 3 days and gradually decline after 3–4 months

        1. Duration depends on area injected, dose, and formulation used.

        2. Repeated injections may lead to an increased response duration.

III. Types and Formulations in North America
    A. Type A for cosmetic and therapeutic applications
        1. OnabotulinumtoxinA (Botox®/Botox® Cosmetic Allergan, Irvine, CA).
        2. AbobotulinumtoxinA (Dysport®, Medicis, Scottsdale, AZ).
        3. IncobotulinumtoxinA (Xeomin®, Merz Pharmaceuticals, Frankfurt Am Main, Germany).
        4. PrabotulinumtoxinA (Jeuveau®, Evolus, Santa Barbara, CA).
    B. Type B for therapeutic applications
        1. RimabotulinumtoxinB (Myobloc®/Neurobloc® Solstice Neuroscience, Malvern, PA).
IV. Cosmetic Indications and Uses[2] (Table 15.1 and Figure 15.1)
    A. Approved by the Food and Drug Administration (FDA)
        1. Glabellar rhytides (frown lines).
        2. Forehead lines.
        3. Lateral canthal lines (Crow's feet).
    B. Off-label uses
        1. Hyperkinetic lines in the upper and lower face and neck.
        2. Eyebrow elevation ("chemical brow lift").
        3. Restoration of facial symmetry and balance.
        4. Widening of the eyes.
        5. Sculpting the jaw.
        6. Adjunct to other cosmetic procedures to enhance and prolong the results.
            a. Soft-tissue augmentation (fillers).
            b. Laser and light-based therapies.
            c. Plastic surgery.

> The only current FDA-approved cosmetic uses of botulinum (e.g., Botox®) are for glabellar rhytides (frown lines), horizontal forehead lines, and lateral canthal lines (crow's feet).

TABLE 15.1

On- and Off-Label Treatment Indications in the Face and Neck for Botulinum Neurotoxin Type A

Indications	Target Muscle
Glabellar frown lines	Corrugator supercilii, procerus, orbicularis oculi, depressor supercilii (medial fibers of orbicularis oculi inserting into dermis)
Horizontal forehead lines	Frontalis
Lateral canthal lines (crow's feet)	Lateral fibers of orbicularis oculi
Bunny lines and nasal flare	Procerus, superior transverse nasalis
Nasolabial folds	Levator labii superioris alaeque nasi (lateral belly)
Nose tip depression	Depressor nasii septi
Vertical perioral rhytides (smoker's lines or bar code lines)	Orbicularis oris
Gummy smile	Levator labii superioris alaeque nasi (lateral belly), depressor nasii septi
Downturned mouth	Depressor anguli oris
Marionette or howdy doody lines (melomental folds)	Depressor anguli oris
Mental crease	Mentalis and depressor labii inferioris
Peau d'orange chin (dimpled, pebbly appearance)	Mentalis
Horizontal necklace lines	Platysma
Platysmal vertical bands	Platysma

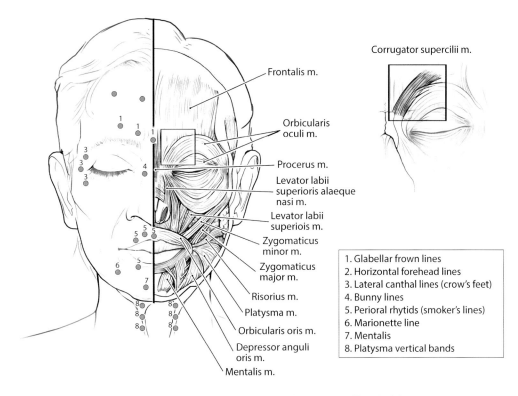

Corrugator supercilii m.

Frontalis m.

Orbicularis oculi m.

Procerus m.

Levator labii superioris alaeque nasi m.

Levator labii superiois m.

Zygomaticus minor m.

Zygomaticus major m.

Risorius m.

Platysma m.

Orbicularis oris m.

Depressor anguli oris m.

Mentalis m.

1. Glabellar frown lines
2. Horizontal forehead lines
3. Lateral canthal lines (crow's feet)
4. Bunny lines
5. Perioral rhytids (smoker's lines)
6. Marionette line
7. Mentalis
8. Platysma vertical bands

FIGURE 15.1 Common neurotoxin injection sites (left) and underlying muscles affected (right).

V. Therapeutic (noncosmetic) Indications and Uses

   A. Approved by the FDA

     1. Strabimus.

     2. Blepharospasm.

     3. Hemifacial spasm.

     4. Cervical dystonia.

     5. Axillary hyperhidrosis/palmar hyperhidrosis.

     6. Chronic migraine.

     7. Urinary incontinence.

   B. Off-label uses

     1. Lower urinary tract disorders.

     2. Gastrointestinal tract disorders.

     3. Spasticity.

     4. Spasmodic dysphonia.

     5. Sialorrhea.

     6. Temporomandibular disorder.

     7. Chronic musculoskeletal pain.

     8. Diabetic neuropathy.

     9. Postherpetic trigeminal neuralgia.

     10. Wound healing and treatment of scars.

VI. Adverse Effects and Complications[3]

RECONSTITUTING A 100 UNIT VIAL OF BOTOX

Add 2.5 cc of normal saline to produce 4 units per 0.1 cc.

A. Contraindications

1. Peripheral motor neuropathic disease (e.g., myasthenia gravis) and multiple sclerosis have increased risk of systemic side effects.

2. Calcium channel blockers, aminoglycoside antibiotics, and cyclosporine may potentiate neurotoxin effects.

B. Injection-related (transient) side effects

1. Swelling.

2. Bruising.

3. Pain.

C. Complications

1. Diffusion into nontargeted or glandular tissue in surrounding areas.

   a. Overenthusiastic doses.

   b. Inappropriate injection sites.

   c. Poor injection technique.

Although seemingly easy to inject botulinum toxin, serious complications can occur. These complications can be minimized when injections are performed by physicians who have had extensive anatomic training and experience.

2. Upper face.

   a. Ptosis (brow or eyelid). May treat with apraclonidine 0.5% ophthalmic solution (Iopidine) t.i.d. to affected eye. Will result in 1–2 mm of temporary eyelid elevation. Apraclonidine is an alpha-2 adrenergic agonist that causes Müller muscles to contract.

   b. Epiphora.

   c. Diplopia.

   d. Dry eye.

   e. Asymmetrical brows.

3. Lower face.

   a. Flaccid cheek.

   b. Asymmetrical smile.

   c. Incompetent mouth.

   d. Dysphagia.

   e. Weakness of neck flexors.

D. Clinical safety record

1. Strong safety record with cosmetic use.[4]

2. Serious adverse events more common with much higher therapeutic doses.[5]

Conclusion

In cosmetic dermatology, botulinum toxin not only reduces the appearance of fine lines and folds, but also can be used toward more artful outcomes, such as shaping and sculpting the face. While minor side effects can and do occur, serious complications tend to occur in association with high therapeutic doses. Over 20 years of data support the efficacy and clinical safety of botulinum neurotoxin when used by experienced physicians in appropriate doses.

REFERENCES

1. Carruthers A, Carruthers J. Botulinum Toxin Type A: History and Current Cosmetic Use in the Upper Face. Semin Cutan Med Surg 2001; 20: 71–84.

2. Carruthers J, Carruthers A. Botulinum Toxin in Facial Rejuvenation: An Update. Dermatol Clin 2009; 27: 417–425.
3. Klein AW. Complications, Adverse Reactions, and Insights With the Use of Botulinum Toxin. Dermatol Surg 2003; 29: 549–556.
4. Carruthers J, Carruthers A. Complications of Botulinum Toxin A. Facial Plast Surg Clin North Am 2007; 15: 51–54.
5. Cote TR, Mohan AK, Polder JA, Walton MK, Braun MM. Botulinum Toxin Type A Injections: Adverse Events Reported to the US Food and Drug Administration in Therapeutic and Cosmetic Cases. J Am Acad Dermatol 2005; 53: 407–415.

16

Soft Tissue Fillers

Jeanette M. Black and Derek H. Jones

Introduction

Many injectable filler products have become available to be used as volume replacement for age-associated atrophy and correction of wrinkles or folds. The popularity of temporary injectable fillers continues to grow as new filler substances enter the market and the indications for use expand. The diversity of injectable fillers offers the physician many options to tailor treatment to each individual's needs. Injectable fillers are safe, predictable, and effective when used by an experienced physician injector for cosmetic enhancement in a properly selected patient. Since there is a significant potential for adverse events, an understanding of how to prevent and treat adverse events is paramount.

I. Patient Preparation
   A. Counsel the patient
      1. Educate patients about underlying anatomy and normal age-related changes.[1]
      2. Review the inherent complication risks and potential downtime.[2]
      3. Discuss the cost, expectations, and longevity of fillers.[3]
   B. Physical examination of the patient[1]
      1. Evaluate the patient for baseline asymmetry and subjective defects and document with photographs.
      2. Procedures should be deferred if there are any preexisting skin conditions in the treatment area such as seborrheic dermatitis, impetigo, or herpetic ulcerations.
   C. Patient preparation
      1. Patients should abstain from nonessential medications that could inhibit platelet function and lead to increased bleeding and ecchymosis (aspirin, nonsteroidal anti-inflammatory drugs [NSAIDS], omega-3 fatty acids, fish oil, and many over-the-counter supplements).[1]
      2. Consider herpes simplex prophylaxis for lip augmentation in patients with a history of recurrent cold sores.[4]
      3. Contraindications include prior allergy to filler material or its constituents (e.g., lidocaine).[2]

      Although the FDA has approved specific indications for certain fillers, this process is continually evolving and changes yearly.

      4. Obtain informed consent.
         a. Know the Food and Drug Administration (FDA)-approved indications as many uses of injectable fillers are considered "off-label".[5]
         b. Document that the patient understands all risks, indications, benefits, and options of the injectable fillers being used.[3]

D. The patient should be positioned comfortably, usually seated upright, and in such a way that gravity-dependent defects are not obscured. Lying the patient flat distorts facial contours[1]

   1. Adequate lighting.

   2. During injection, tilting the patient slightly recumbent creates more comfort for both the physician and patient.

E. Clean technique[1]

   1. Prepare the skin by swabbing the treatment site with isopropyl alcohol, chloroxylenol, or chlorhexidine. Note that chlorhexidine should be avoided near the eyes and ears.

   2. Change gloves and needles after intraoral manipulation or injection.

F. Anesthesia[4,5]

   1. Ice or cold packs.

   2. Topical anesthetics prior to filler injections.

     a. Preparations containing lidocaine, tetracaine, benzocaine, and prilocaine (Table 10.2).

   3. Nerve blocks with 2% lidocaine.

   4. Injectable fillers are often premixed with lidocaine (Table 16.1).

II. Injection Techniques[1]

A. Serial puncture (Figure 16.1A)

   1. Small amounts of filler are sequentially deposited closely together along the wrinkle or fold, and postinjection massage is used to help distribute the filler.

TABLE 16.1

FDA Approved Fillers 2018

Hyaluronic Acid	Manufacturer	G'[e]	Composition
Restylane®[a]	Galderma	Medium	Hyaluronic acid
Restylane® Defyne	Galderma	Medium	Hyaluronic acid
Restylane® Refyne	Galderma	Low	Hyaluronic acid
Restylane Silk®[b]	Galderma	Medium	Hyaluronic acid
Restylane® Lyft[b] (formerly Perlane®)	Galderma	Medium	Hyaluronic acid
Juvéderm®[c]	Allergan		Hyaluronic acid
Juvéderm® Ultra[c]	Allergan	Low	Hyaluronic acid
Juvéderm® Ultra Plus[c]	Allergan	Low	Hyaluronic acid
Juvéderm Vobella®[c]	Allergan	Low medium	Hyaluronic acid
Juvéderm Vollure™[c]	Allergan	Medium	Hyaluronic acid
Juvéderm Voluma®[c]	Allergan	Medium	Hyaluronic acid
Revanesse® Versa™[d]	Prollenium Medical Technologies	Low	Hyaluronic acid
Belotero Balance®	Merz Aesthetics	Low	Hyaluronic acid
Nonhyaluronic Acid	**Manufacturer**		**Composition**
Radiesse®[d]	Merz Aesthetics	High	Calcium hydroxylapatite
Bellafill®(formerly Artefill®)[b]	Suneva Medical		Poly methyl methacrylate (PMMA) microspheres and bovine collagen
Sculptra®	Galderma		Poly-L-lactic acid
Silikon®	Alcon Labs		Dimethylpolysiloxane

[a] Also available as "L" that contains 0.3% lidocaine.
[b] With lidocaine.
[c] Also available as "XC" (extra comfort) product with lidocaine.
[d] Also available as (+) that contains 0.3% lidocaine.
[e] G' is a measure of how easily a material can be deformed with opposing force.

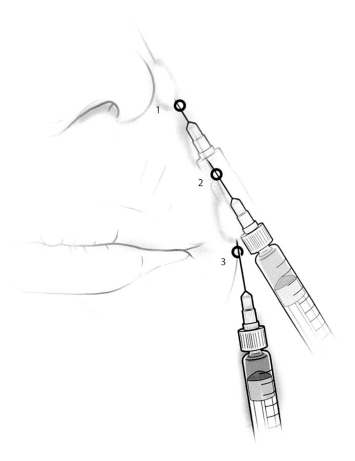

FIGURE 16.1A   Serial puncture technique. Several filler injections are separately performed along a crease or wrinkle line.

    B. Linear threading (Figure 16.1B)

        1. Continuous deposition of filler as the needle tip is pulled backward in a retrograde direction. This type of deposition can also be done in an anterograde direction.

    C. Fanning (Figure 16.1C)

        1. Multiple threading injections in different directions without withdrawing the needle from the original insertion site.

    D. Cross-hatching or radial injection (Figure 16.1D)

        1. Evenly spaced linear injections in a grid-like pattern.

    E. Depot

        1. The deep injection of a large amount of filler that lasts a long time.

        2. Depot injections are followed by postinjection massage to blend the filler into the natural contour of the region.

    F. Blunt-tipped cannulas can be used to minimize inadvertent vascular injury and intravascular injection

        1. Cannulas are advised for injections into the cheek area medial to the mid-pupillary line.

III. Common Treatment Locations[3]

    A. Upper face: temple, brow, forehead

    B. Midface: cheek, lid-cheek junction, tear trough, nasolabial fold, radial/lateral cheek and eyelid lines, superficial static fine ("etched-in") lines, and atrophic acne scars

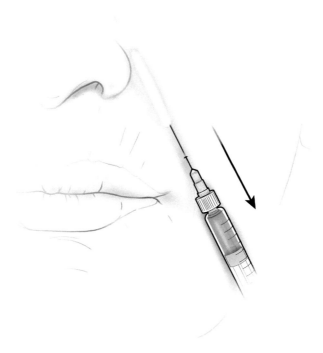

FIGURE 16.1B Linear threading technique. Continuous filler injection during needle withdrawal.

      C. Lower face: marionette lines, chin, and mandibular line
      D. Lips
      E. Dorsal hands
    IV. Treatment depth: extremely important to safely produce desired result. The selection of the appropriate filler for a chosen depth is dependent upon several factors, the most important of

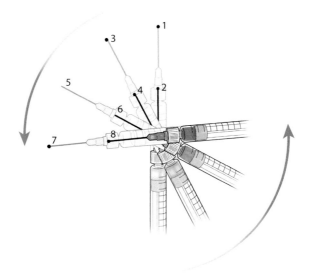

FIGURE 16.1C Fanning technique. After a single injection of the needle, the filler is injected by threading in different directions.

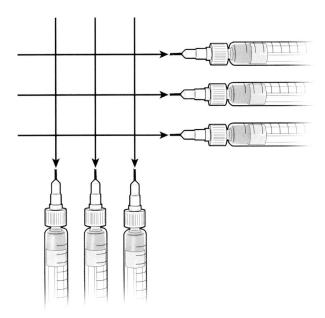

FIGURE 16.1D   Cross-hatching injection technique. Deposition of filler by linear threading in a grid-like pattern.

which are filler viscosity and elasticity. Fillers with high viscosity and elasticity have a firmer feel, spread less, and tend to remain where they are injected and allow for precise sculpting. A low viscosity and elasticity filler tends to spread into tissue and have a softer feel. The elasticity property of a filler is expressed as the G prime (elastic modulus). The higher the G prime (G'), the less it deforms under pressure and the lower the G', the more it deforms under pressure[6]

A.   Superficial (intradermal)[1]

    1.   For very superficial static fine ("etched-in") wrinkles. These lines include horizontal forehead lines, radial/lateral cheek and eyelid lines, and vertical lip lines.

    2.   Hyaluronic acid (HA) fillers for this purpose have a low G'.

Generally, the viscosity and elasticity of a filler are related to the recommended depth of its injection. A filler with low viscosity and low elasticity is best placed more superficially.

B.   Intermediate (subcutaneous layer)[1]

    1.   The most common injection plane.

    2.   Suitable for moderate to deep wrinkles and folds and subcutaneous volumizing.

    3.   HA fillers for this purpose have a medium G'.

    4.   Most safely performed with a blunt-tipped cannula that may help prevent accidental intravascular injection or vascular injury.

C.   Deep (periosteal level)[1]

    1.   Most suitable for volumizing of the temple, zygomatic cheek area, chin, and mandible.

    2.   HA fillers for this purpose have a high G'.

    3.   Periosteal injections should be performed with caution where named blood vessels may emanate deep near bone, such as the medial cheek (infraorbital artery) and the central mandible (facial artery).

V.   Filler Types (see Table 16.1)

A.   HA derivatives (Restylane Lyft®, Restylane®, Restylane Silk®, Restylane Defyne®, Restylane Refyne®, Juvéderm Voluma®, Juvéderm Vollure®, Juvéderm Volbella®, Juvéderm UltraPlus®, Juvéderm Ultra®, Belotero Balance®, Revanesse Versa®)[1,5]

1. HA is a major component of human skin and synovial fluid. In the skin, it is found in the extracellular matrix of connective tissue and declines with age, creating wrinkles, folds, and volume loss.

2. HA fillers are derived from streptococcal fermentation.

3. HAs are the most widely used injectable fillers with a variety of indications. HA is viscoelastic and immunologically inert.

4. HAs are the only fillers that are immediately reversible ("erasable") with injectable hyaluronidase, which is derived from bacterial (Streptococcus) fermentation.

5. Cross-linking modifications impart different attributes to each HA product. Cross-linking creates macromolecules that are larger and more stable than natural HA. As cross-linking increases, liquid is converted to a gel. In general, the greater the degree of cross-linking, the greater the resistance to tissue degradation.

6. When injected, HA filler binds water. Overtime, as HA degrades, it binds more and more water but its overall volume stays the same (isovolumetric degradation).

7. The molecular weight, concentration, and amount of cross-linking of HA products affect the longevity and the ideal injection depth for fine to medium to deep wrinkles and folds.

8. Products used for volumizing lips, nasolabial* folds, cheeks, temples, tear troughs, chin, mandibles, dorsal hands, and superficial static fine ("etched-in") wrinkles.

9. Restylane Lyft® (formerly known as Perlane®).

    a. HA approved for deep dermal injection to correct moderate to severe facial folds and wrinkles, such as nasolabial folds, age-related midface volume loss, and volume deficits of the dorsal hands.

    There are numerous HA fillers, some with and some without lidocaine.

10. Restylane®.

    a. FDA approved for mid to deep dermal injection to treat moderate to severe wrinkles and folds, such as nasolabial folds and for lip augmentation in patients over the age of 21.

11. Restylane Defyne®.

    a. FDA approved for the correction of moderate to severe deep facial wrinkles and folds, such as nasolabial folds.

12. Restylane Refyne®.

    a. FDA approved for the correction of moderate to severe facial wrinkles and folds, such as nasolabial folds.

13. Restylane Silk®.

    a. FDA approved for lip augmentation and dermal implantation for correction of perioral rhytides in patients over the age of 21.

14. Juvéderm Voluma®.

    a. FDA approved for deep subcutaneous or supraperiosteal injection for cheek augmentation to correct age-related volume deficit in the midface in patients over the age of 21.

15. Juvéderm Vollure®.

    a. FDA approved for injection into the mid to deep dermis for correction of moderate to severe facial wrinkles and folds, such as nasolabial folds.

---

* In this chapter, the term nasolabial is used rather than melolabial as this term is used by the FDA. Technically, melolabial fold refers to the fold between the cheek and the lip, whereas nasolabial fold refers to the fold between the nose and the lip. Because of inaccurate conventional usage, the adjectival terms nasolabial and melolabial are used synonymously.

16. Juvéderm Vobella®.
    a. FDA approved for lip augmentation and for correction of perioral rhytides.
17. Juvéderm UltraPlus®.
    a. FDA approved for mid to deep dermal injections to correct moderate to severe facial wrinkles, such as nasolabial folds.
18. Juvéderm Ultra®.
    a. FDA approved for mid to deep dermal injections to correct moderate to severe facial wrinkles, such as nasolabial folds.
19. Belotero Balance®.
    a. FDA approved for injection into facial tissue to smooth wrinkles and folds, especially around the nose and mouth.
20. Revanesse® Versa™.
    a. FDA approved for injection of moderate to severe wrinkles and creases, such as nasolabial folds.

B. Poly-L-lactic acid (Sculptra®)[1]
    1. Powdered lyophilized polyglactin 910 (the same synthetic compound used to make Vicryl® suture) reconstituted with sterile water 24 hours or more prior to injection.
    2. Stimulates fibroblasts to produce collagen.
    3. FDA approved for use in shallow to deep nasolabial fold contour deficiencies and other facial wrinkles and for the correction of HIV facial lipoatrophy.
    4. Useful for HIV lipoatrophy and volume augmentation.
    5. Initially, microspheres add volume (thus a volumizer). Overtime, the microspheres are engulfed and metabolized by macrophages to produce lactic acid, carbon dioxide, and water.
    6. Postinjection massages are recommended to prevent granuloma formation.
        a. Typically, patients are instructed to massage the treatment area for 5 minutes, 5 times a day for 5 days ("Rule of 5s").
    7. A series of monthly treatments (usually three) are needed for optimal correction.
    8. Red nodules may appear 7–12 months after injection associated with idiopathic immune response.

C. Calcium hydroxylapatite (Radiesse®)[1]
    1. Commonly used for moderate to severe folds, cheek volumizing, HIV facial lipoatrophy, and hand rejuvenation.
    2. Calcium hydroxylapatite microspheres suspended in a polysaccharide carrier (glycerin and sodium carboxy methyl cellulose) that is absorbed. The microspheres stay in place and activate fibroblasts to produce collagen.
    3. Injected deeply at the dermal-subcutaneous junction.
    4. FDA approved for subdermal implantation to treat moderate to severe facial wrinkles and folds, such as nasolabial folds, and to correct volume loss in the dorsum of the hands.[5]
    5. Contraindicated for lip augmentation as calcium hydroxylapatite is opaque and mucosal lumps may form.
    6. The product is radio-opaque and may be visible on radiographs and CT scans.[1]

D. Highly purified silicone oil (polydimethylsiloxane) (Silikon® 1000)[1]
    1. Best employed off-label for severe HIV-associated facial lipoatrophy.
    2. Deposited using a microdroplet serial puncture technique.
    3. Permanent.
    4. FDA approved only for use as an injectable intraocular tamponade for retinal detachment.

E. Polymethylmethacrylate (PMMA) microspheres (Bellafill® formerly known as Artefill®)[1]

1. PMMA microspheres suspended in bovine collagen and lidocaine.

2. Contains bovine collagen and therefore requires prior skin testing to screen for hypersensitivity reactions.

3. Used for structural contouring and deep wrinkles and folds.

4. As the bovine collagen portion is degraded, the remaining PMMA microspheres stimulate fibroblasts that encapsulate and keep the microspheres in place.

5. Permanent.

6. FDA approved to treat moderate to severe nasolabial folds in patients over the age of 21 and to improve the appearance of acne scars.

F. Lipotransfer[1,2,7]

1. Autologous donor fat harvested from the patient's abdomen using a 12–14 gauge microliposuction cannula. May be done with tumescent or nontumescent anesthesia.

2. Before it is injected, the adipose tissue is washed with normal saline and inverted or centrifuged to separate blood and liquid fat from solid fat. The blood and liquid fat are decanted leaving only solid fat.

3. The separated solid fat is injected with a spinal tap needle using retrograde technique.

4. Harvested fat can be stored frozen for up to 12–18 months.

5. Used for deep facial volumetric correction and hand rejuvenation.

6. Great variability of duration of correction, but can possibly be permanent.

7. Usually requires multiple (usually three) injection sessions.

VI. Complications[1]

A. Erythema, swelling, pain, and ecchymosis are common treatment site responses

1. Generally, resolves within 1 week without treatment.

2. To reduce risk of ecchymosis.

   a. Abstain from nonessential platelet inhibiting medications 7–10 days prior to treatment.

   b. Avoid vigorous exercise for 24 hours after treatment.

   c. Using a blunt-tipped cannula helps to avoid vascular injury.

   d. Bruising can be treated with intense pulse light, pulse dye laser, or potassium titanyl phosphate (KTP) laser that rapidly breaks down red cells in tissue, which create the bruise.

B. More serious complications include contour irregularities, nodules, Tyndall effect (blue-grey discoloration due to scattering of shorter wavelength blue light and transmission of other, longer wavelengths; associated with superficial injections of HA filler), granuloma formation, bacterial biofilms, hypersensitivity reactions, and vascular occlusion

C. HA derivatives can be degraded with injectable hyaluronidase (Vitrase®, Hylenex®)

Vascular occlusion, although rare, can occur with inadvertent filler injection into an artery in a highly vascular area.

1. Consider skin testing of hyaluronidase in those with history of anaphylaxis to hymenoptera stings (yellow jackets and honey bees) due to theoretical cross-reactivity.

D. Vascular occlusion is an emergency and should be treated immediately

1. Warning signs include immediate or delayed blanching, excessive pain, duskiness, and reticulated erythema, which may herald severe tissue necrosis.

   a. Immediately discontinue injection if warning signs occur.

b. Highest risk area for ulceration or necrosis is glabellar area. One needs to be particularly careful to aspirate prior to injection in this area.

2. Treatments include hyaluronidase, warm compression, massage, topical nitroglycerin paste, and aspirin while use of prednisone, hyperbaric oxygen, and low-molecular-weight heparin have been reported with variable results.

3. Accidental intravascular injection and filler embolization may lead to irreversible blindness, ophthalmoplegia, and stroke.

a. Prevented by thorough understanding of anatomy in the high-risk area of the central face where vascular communication exists between the supratrochlear, supraorbital, dorsal nasal, and angular artery with the retinal circulation.

b. Can be avoided by aspiration prior to each injection to ensure that the injection needle is not within a blood vessel.

c. Ocular pain and visual impairment require emergency evaluation by an ophthalmologist.

d. Neurologic symptoms require an emergency evaluation by a neurologist.

Conclusion

Physicians must keep abreast of advancements in injection techniques and indications as novel injectable filler products become available. A combination of multiple injectable fillers may be necessary to achieve optimal results. Filler substance injection can also be combined with other cosmetic procedures such as laser resurfacing, chemodenervation (e.g., Botox® injections), and chemical peeling for maximum benefit. It is crucial to use proper technique and surgical skill to achieve the best outcomes and avoid potential complications.

REFERENCES

1. Jones D, Bacigalupi R, Beleznay K. Injectable soft tissue augmentation. In: Dermatology. 4th edition (Bolognia JL, Schaffer J, Cerroni L, editors). Mosby Elsevier, Philadelphia, 2017; pp. 2649–2660.
2. Alam M, Gladstone H, Kramer EM et al. ASDS Guidelines of Care: Injectable Fillers. Dermatol Surg 2008; 34: S115–S148.
3. Jones D, Editor. Injectabe Fillers: Principles and Practice. Wiley Blackwell, Hoboken, NJ, 2010.
4. Mariwalla K, Leffell DJ. Primer in Dermatologic Surgery: A Study Companion. 2nd Edition. American Society for Dermatologic Surgery, Rolling Meadows, IL, 2011; pp. 109–114.
5. Food and Drug Administration. "Dermal Fillers (Soft Tissue Fillers)." 3 March 2021, www.fda.gov/medical-devices/aesthetic-cosmetic-devices/dermal-fillers-soft-tissue-fillers#:~:text=Dermal%20fillers%2C%20also%20known%20as,the%20edges%20of%20the%20mouth)%2C.
6. Sundaram H, Voigts B, Beer K, Meland M. Comparison of the Rheological Properties of Viscosity and Elasticity in Two Categories of Soft Tissue Fillers: Calcium Hydroxylapatite and Hyaluronic Acid. Derm Surg 2010; 36: 1859–1865.
7. Donofrio LM. Structural Autologous Lipoaugmentation: A Pan-Facial Technique. Dermatol Surg 2000; 26: 1129–1134.

17

Chemical Peeling

Gary D. Monheit

Introduction

Chemical peeling remains an important method to even out skin pigmentation and irregularities mostly related to chronic sun damage. Although the technique of chemical peeling is relatively simple, selection of patients and peeling agents is critical to achieve optimal results.

I. Chemical peeling: the topical application of a chemical or combination of chemicals to the skin surface to intentionally create injury to a specific depth. This destruction promotes skin exfoliation and peeling followed by growth of "rejuvenated" skin, i.e., new epidermis and superficial dermis

   A. Longstanding safety and efficacy record

   B. Easy to perform

   C. Low cost

   D. Requires short postprocedure downtime but dependent on peel depth

II. Peeling agents are classified as (very) superficial, medium, and deep based on their level of penetration/depth of injury (Table 17.1)

   A. Superficial: epidermal injury only

   B. Medium: injury through epidermis into papillary dermis (0.45–0.6 mm in depth)

   C. Deep: injury through epidermis, papillary dermis, and into upper reticular dermis (0.6–0.8 mm in depth)

III. Seven major indications for a chemical peeling

   A. To improve the appearance and to smooth out actinically (sun-damaged) skin

   B. To reduce or eliminate rhytides (skin wrinkles)

   C. To flatten mild scarring (e.g., acne scarring)

   D. To destroy epidermal lesions (e.g., actinic keratoses, lentigines)

   E. To improve underlying skin diseases such as acne

   F. To remove pigmentary dyschromias

   G. To blend the effects of other resurfacing procedures, such as dermabrasion or laserabrasion

IV. In general, the degree of skin surface irregularity is proportional to the depth of chemical peel required to reach the desired endpoint

V. Healing and downtime postprocedure are dependent on the depth of the peel

   A. Superficial: 1–2 days

   B. Medium: 5–10 days

   C. Deep: 10–14 days

TABLE 17.1

Variables Associated with Peel Depth

	Superficial	Medium Depth	Deep
Indications	Mild photoaging, mild acne, melasma	Superficial wrinkles, moderate actinic damage	Deep wrinkles
Depth	Epidermis	Epidermis and papillary dermis	Epidermis/papillary dermis, upper reticular dermis
Frosting	No[a]	Yes	Yes
Common agents	Glycolic acid, TCA 10%–20%, tretinoin, Jessner solution[b]	35% TCA + Jessner solution[b] or glycolic acid 70% or CO_2 slush	Baker-Gordon formula[c]
Complications	None	Hyperpigmentation, scarring	Hypopigmentation, cardiotoxicity
Number of treatment sessions	6–8	1	1
Downtime	1–2 days	5–10 days	10–14 days

[a] If "frosting" occurs, it is considered to be pseudofrosting as it can be easily wiped off.
[b] Resorcinol (14 g), salicylic acid (14 g), lactic acid (14 g), ethanol 95% (up to 100 mL).
[c] 88% phenol (3 cc), distilled water (2 cc), septisol liquid soap (8 drops), croton oil (3 drops).

VI. Preoperative Consultation

    A. To determine patient cosmetic concerns/goals

        1. Can peel satisfy patient's desired result or are other modalities also needed (fillers, toxins, lasers, etc.)?

    B. To assess patient skin type: Fitzpatrick skin type (I–VI), Glogau classification (I–IV) (see Tables 2.1 and 2.2)

        1. Fitzpatrick types IV–VI are at particular risk of dyschromia postprocedure.

        2. All skin types require daily broad-spectrum sunscreen before and after peeling to reduce risk of postoperative hyperpigmentation.

    C. To determine previous resurfacing, facial surgery, or medications that may adversely affect a chemical peel (especially medium, deep peels). These include systemic isotretinoin therapy within the last year

    D. To obtain history of herpes simplex virus (HSV) or abnormal scarring, keloids

        1. Antiviral prophylaxis not needed for superficial peels; recommended for all medium and deep peels regardless of HSV history.

        2. To discuss patient consent, cost, and expected downtime.

        3. To explain limitations and potential side effects.

VII. Preoperative Skin Care Regimen

    A. Sun avoidance and sunscreen application: to reduce baseline pigmentation and reduce potential postprocedure pigmentation

    B. Retinoids: pretreatment with topical retinoids for 6 weeks prepeel accelerates healing, decreases downtime, and increases peel depth. Topical retinoids are discontinued 48 hours prior to peel

    C. Bleaching agents (controversial): use before and after peel may minimize risk of postpeel hyperpigmentation, especially in Fitzpatrick skin types III or higher

VIII. Superficial Chemical Peels (Table 17.2)

    A. Cause partial to full-thickness epidermal injury; no injury to the dermis

    B. Indications: mild photoaging, mild inflammatory acne, rosacea, lentigines, ephelides (freckles), melasma, postinflammatory hyperpigmentation

TABLE 17.2

Superficial Peeling Agents

Agent	Indications	Actions	White Frosting	Neutralization
Trichloroacetic acid 10%–25% (TCA)	Photoaging	Protein precipitation	Yes	Unnecessary
Jessner's solution[a]	Photoaging, melasma	Breaks intercellular bridges	No	Unnecessary
Salicylic acid	Acne, photoaging	Keratolytic, comedolytic	Yes	Unnecessary
Solid CO_2 slush	Acne	Cellular dehydration with necrosis	No	Unnecessary
α-hydroxy acid 20%–70% (AHA)	Lentigos, melasma	Keratolytic (low concentration), epidermolytic (high concentration)	No	Yes (sodium bicarbonate or water)
Tretinoin solution	Photoaging, acne	Desquammation	No	Unnecessary

[a] Resorcinol (14 g), salicylic acid (14 g), lactic acid (14 g), ethanol 95% (up to 100 mL).

C. Usually requires six to eight peels weekly or every other week to achieve desired result
   1. Improvements often subtle with photoaged skin.
   2. Minimal appreciable effect on deep wrinkles, furrows.
D. Very light peeling agents: low-concentration glycolic acid (α-hydroxy acid), trichloroacetic acid (TCA) 10%–20%, Jessner's solution, tretinoin, salicylic acid (β-hydroxy acid). Jessner's solution is resorcinol (14 g), salicylic acid (14 g), lactic acid (14 g), in ethanol 95% (up to 100 mL)
E. Light peeling agents: 70% glycolic acid, 15–25% TCA, solid CO_2 slush (solid carbon dioxide wrapped in a towel and dipped in a 3:1 solution of acetone and alcohol, respectively)
F. Recommended that glycolic acid be neutralized with water after 2–4 minutes
G. Salicyclic acid may cause perifollicular frosting because it is lipophilic and concentrates in the pilosebaceous units. This reagent is preferred for acne
H. Very light and light peeling agents usually do not result in frosting or peeling (desquamation)
I. Salicylic acid peel is avoided in patients with strawberry allergy
J. Postpeel downtime/healing: 1–4 days (very light peels, no downtime)
K. Repetitive "maintenance" peels are the rule to maintain results
L. Net effect of repetitive superficial peels never approaches degree of benefit seen with a single medium or deep peel
M. Routine postpeel antibiotic and antiviral are NOT required with superficial chemical peels
N. Postpeel routine includes sun avoidance, thin coat of petrolatum, or antibiotic ointment

IX. Medium-Depth Chemical Peels
   A. Injury (coagulation necrosis) to the papillary dermis, occasionally upper reticular dermis (dependent on the agent used, concentration used, and application time)
   B. Indications: moderate actinic damage, dyschromias, superficial rhytides, scars, epidermal hyperkeratotic lesions (e.g., actinic keratoses, seborrheic keratoses)
   C. Can also be used to "blend" or transition the periphery of deeper resurfacing procedures

    D. Historically, TCA 50% was the gold standard medium-depth agent

       1. Results were unpredictable.

       2. Complications were scarring and hyperpigmentation.

    E. Recently, a variety of medium-depth peels using a combination of agents has led to more consistent results and fewer postpeel complications

       1. Common medium-depth peel combinations include: Jessner's/TCA 35% (Monheit peel[1]), glycolic acid 70%/TCA 35%, solid CO_2/TCA 35%.

       2. The common objective of these combination peels is to cause mild epidermal injury with application of the first agent, followed by deeper, uniform, controlled penetration of the second agent, TCA 35%.

> Medium-depth chemical peels usually combine 35% TCA with another peeling agent such as Jessner's or glycolic acid.

    F. Depth of peel can be assessed by the amount of skin whitening or "frosting" noted after application of the TCA. Frost is a visible indication of precipitated protein coagulation and cannot be easily wiped off. Pseudofrosting implies a crystallization of the peeling agent that can be wiped off. Often happens with salicylic acid chemical peels. Levels of frosting

       1. Level I: frosting with streaky surface whitening.

       2. Level II: frosting with erythema showing through.

       3. Level III: frosting with little or no background erythema (indicates peel extends through papillary dermis).

    G. Depth of peel is dependent on whether skin degreased before peel, peeling agent concentration, and number of applications (passes) during peel session

    H. Medium-depth peels for epidermal growths such as actinic keratoses not only improve the burden of photodamage immediately but have also been shown to reduce the incidence of future nonmelanoma skin cancers in treated areas

    I. Postpeel downtime is 5–10 days; erythema/edema are common soon after the peel, followed by superficial epidermal darkening and "paint-chipped" desquamation

    J. Collagen remodeling occurs over a 3- to 4-month period

    K. Antiviral prophylaxis is recommended in all patients, regardless of previous HSV history, to be continued for 10–14 days after the peel

    L. Postpeel sun avoidance/sunscreen use is crucial to avoid hyperpigmentation

 X. Deep Chemical Peels

    A. Injury to the epidermis, papillary dermis, and upper reticular dermis, inducing new collagen

    B. Indicated for advanced photodamage

    C. Phenol peels

       1. Baker-Gordon peel solution.

          a. Combination of phenol 88% (3 mL), distilled water (2 mL), septisol liquid soap (8 drops), and croton oil (3 drops). Concentration of phenol is reduced from 88% to 50% or 55% by the croton oil.

       2. Hetter peel solution.

          a. Same ingredients as the Baker-Gordon peel solution above but varies in phenol and croton oil concentration so that the intensity of the peel can be decreased.[2]

    D. Phenol is cardiotoxic, hepatotoxic, and nephrotoxic

    E. Full-face procedures need to be performed over a 60- to 90-minute period of time to prevent systemic absorption of phenol and limit systemic complications

1. Intravenous hydration with Lactated Ringer's solution or normal saline before and during the peel helps to keep systemic phenol levels low and minimize toxicity.
2. Continuous blood pressure, pulse oximetry, and cardiac monitoring for arrhythmias are needed throughout the peel and for 1-hour postpeel.
F. Debridement compresses three times a day with aluminum acetate solution (one packet of Domeboro® powder in one quart of water) and antibiotic ointment to avoid crusting and infection until oozing stops
G. Reepithelialization is complete by 2 weeks, but the skin may remain somewhat erythematous and edematous for up to 3 months after the peel
H. Sun avoidance for up to 6 months
I. Hypopigmentation may result from a deep chemical peel. Therefore, not used in darker skin phototypes
J. Ablative lasers are now more commonly used for treatment of advanced photodamage rather than deep chemical peels, as hypopigmentation is less common

Conclusion

Chemical peels can be used to treat a variety of skin disorders, including acne, dyschromias, photoaging, scarring, and epidermal growths. Peels are generally divided into three categories depending on depth of injury: superficial, medium-depth, and deep peels. Pre- and postpeel skin care regimens are vital for ideal outcomes. Low cost, ease of procedure, and longstanding safety and efficacy records make chemical peels useful tools in the dermatologic surgeon's armamentarium, despite the advent of modern lasers and radiofrequency devices.

REFERENCES

1. Monheit GD. The Jessner's + TCA Peel: Medium-Depth Chemical Peel. J Dermatol Surg Oncol 1989; 15: 945–950.
2. Bensimon RH. Croton Oil Peels. Aesthetic Surg J 2008; 28: 33–45.

18

Lasers

Lisa Y. Xu and Mathew M. Avram

Introduction

LASER is an acronym for light amplification by stimulated emission of radiation, which describes the process by which lasers produce light. Light is composed of energy packets, known as photons. Stimulated emission describes the process by which one light photon stimulates an excited atom to emit another photon with the same energy, wavelength, and phase. Lasers work by pumping many atoms into an excited state, forming a large amount of emitted energy. To accomplish this, a laser consists of three components: (1) the medium (gas, liquid, or solid) that when excited stimulates laser light. The medium determines the wavelength, (2) an energy source that acts like a pump to excite the medium, and (3) a delivery system with mirrors that form an optical conduit that confines the amplified light and delivers it to the skin.

Light
Amplification by
Stimulated
Emission of
Radiation

I. Characteristics of Laser Light[1,2]

    A. Monochromatic – one color because the output consists of a single wavelength of light

    B. Coherent – light waves travel in phase, both in time and space, thus causing amplification

    C. Collimated – parallel light beam that does not diverge; allows laser light to be tightly focused and travel long distances without divergence

II. Skin Optics

    A. Tissue effects occur only when a light photon is absorbed by the target molecule, also known as the *chromophore*. The energy transfer from the photon to the chromophore causes chromophore excitation. The absorbed energy is converted to heat (photothermal effect), which gradually diffuses into the surrounding tissue, resulting in a thermal "tissue effect". Another type of tissue effect occurring mainly with tattoos is a photomechanical effect whereby heating results in thermoelastic expansion leading to acoustic and/or shock waves that in turn lead to fragmentation of tattoo pigment or melanin or rupture and increased permeability of cell membranes

    B. In skin, the most important chromophores are melanin, hemoglobin, and water (Table 18.1 and Figure 18.1)

        1. Melanin – primarily absorbs in the ultraviolet (UV) and visible light range; thus, it functions to protect the skin against sunlight.

        2. Hemoglobin – peak absorptions in the blue (400 nm), green (541 nm), and yellow (577 nm) light range.

        3. Water – main component of collagen and absorbs best beyond near infrared region.

Because it absorbs energy, water is referred to as a "chromophore" although it has no color.

TABLE 18.1

Main Target Chromophores Compared

Target Chromophore	Diameter (μm)	Thermal Relaxation Time[a]
Melanosome	0.5–1.0	20–40 ns
Tattoo pigment	0.5–10	20 ns–3 ms
Blood vessel	30–300	5–30 ms
Melanin in hair follicle	200	20–100 ms

[a] Proportional to target diameter squared.

   C. Laser light entering skin is reflected, scattered, transmitted, or absorbed
      1. Reflection from skin surface <5%.
      2. Scattering affected by wavelength. Long wavelengths scatter less.
      3. Transmission dependent on wavelength penetration depth. Long wavelengths penetrate further than short wavelengths.
      4. Energy absorption depends on chromophore absorption spectrum.

III. Laser Parameters
   A. Wavelength – affects the depth of penetration of light into skin. Laser wavelengths primarily lie in the visible and infrared spectrum (Figure 18.1)
      1. From 400 to 1200 nm, the longer the laser wavelength, the deeper the penetration into tissue.

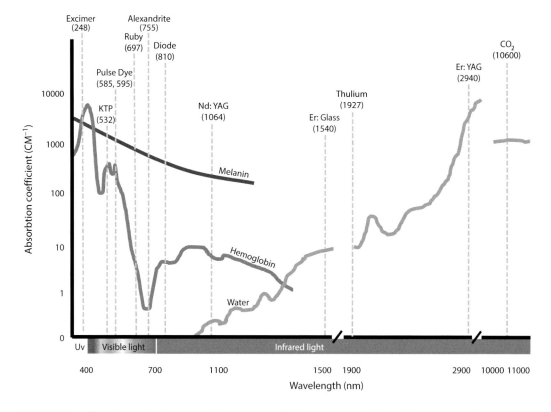

FIGURE 18.1 The relationship between each laser's emitted light wavelength and its relative absorption by the target chromophores of melanin, hemoglobin, and water.

2. Above 1200 nm, water is targeted throughout the dermis and the result is dependent on the degree of tissue destruction. Less tissue destruction occurs around 1500–1900 nm; lasers in this spectrum are considered "non-ablative". More tissue destruction occurs around 3000–10000 nm; lasers in this spectrum are considered "ablative".

Laser parameters that affect depth of penetration:

1. Wavelength
2. Spot size
3. Fluence
4. Pulse duration

B. Spot size – diameter of laser beam on the skin surface, measured in millimeters (mm). A larger spot size decreases laser beam scatter and causes deeper penetration. The spot size also effects fluence and irradiance

C. Fluence – The energy density or amount of energy delivered per unit area, measured in J/cm^2. The local "dose" of laser energy to 1 cm^2 of skin. Should be high enough to damage the target but not too high to destroy the surrounding tissue. Photon energy is proportional to frequency and inversely proportional to wavelength ($E = hf$; $f = c/\lambda$, where E is photon energy, h is the Planck constant, f is the frequency, c is the speed of light, and λ is wavelength). Power (W) is the energy per unit time. Irradiance (power density) is the power per unit area (W/cm^2 or $[J/s]/cm^2$)

D. Pulse duration – duration of the laser pulse (also known as pulse width or exposure time), measured in seconds, milliseconds (10^{-3}), nanoseconds (10^{-9}), or picoseconds (10^{-12}). Must be less than the thermal relaxation time of the target chromophore to minimize damage to surrounding tissue. The shorter the pulse width, the less penetration; the longer the pulse width, the deeper the penetration. Larger structures such as capillaries and hair follicles require longer pulse durations (in the millisecond range for a constant power). Tiny structures such as melanosomes and tattoo pigment require short pulse durations in the nanosecond or picosecond range

1. Laser wave forms – laser light can be released either as continuous, discontinuous, short (pulsed), or very short (Q-switched or mode-locking) modes (Table 18.2). The continuous mode results in more tissue damage than the other modes. The Q (quality)-switched mode uses a shutter to release rapid high-energy short pulses causing rapid heating of the target that produces both a photothermal and photomechanical (shock wave) effect; limits thermal damage to surrounding tissue.

E. Cooling – to prevent burning of the epidermis, some lasers have a cooling feature using cold air

F. Fractionation – laser beam is broken up into microcolumns so that epidermal damage is minimized and subsequent wound healing occurs quickly. The density setting determines the number of microcolumns per unit area of skin

Fractionation of the laser beam is a major advance that speeds wound healing and aids in skin contraction for resurfaced skin.

TABLE 18.2

Laser Wavelengths

	Wavelengths	**Power**	**Example Lasers**
Continuous	Continuous	Low	CO_2
Semicontinuous	Discontinuous	Low	KTP
Pulsed	Short (40–100 ms)	High	Pulsed dye
Q-Switch	Very short (nanosecond)	Very high	QS Nd: YAG
			QS alexandrite (755 nm)
Mode-Locking	Very, very short (picosecond)	Very high	Picosecond alexandrite

treated with a pulse. Subsequent skin tightening occurs with wound contraction of the microcolumns

IV. Theory of Selective Photothermolysis[3,4]
  A. Basis for selection of appropriate laser parameters
  B. Allows for selective heating of the target molecules within a structure such that thermal damage is confined to that structure, with little or no destruction of the surrounding tissue
  C. Requires
     1. Selected wavelength (which also affects its penetration depth) that is preferentially absorbed by the target chromophore.
     2. Energy (J): adjust the energy so fluence (J/cm^2) is high enough to damage the target chromophore but less energy than can cause nonspecific thermal damage.
     3. Pulse duration (pulse width or exposure time) that is shorter than the thermal relaxation time of the target chromophore to confine heat to target structure and not transfer heat to the surrounding structures. When pulse duration is larger than the thermal relaxation time of the target, surrounding tissue is damaged. Expressed in seconds.
  D. *Thermal relaxation time* is defined as the time required for the heated tissue to cool halfway to its initial temperature. Proportional to size of target structure (see Table 18.1)
V. Common Laser Types in Dermatology (see Table 18.3)[5]
VI. Common Uses of Lasers
  A. Hair reduction
     1. Melanin in hair bulge and papilla stem cells is important target chromophores.
     2. Early anagen hair is most susceptible to laser treatments as the hair matrix has the greatest amount of melanin.
     3. Pigmented (black) hairs respond better than grey, blonde, or red hairs.

TABLE 18.3

Common Lasers in Dermatology

Laser	Wavelength (nm)	Medium Source	Target Chromophore	Applications
KTP	532	Crystal	Hemoglobin	Superficial small vessels, superficial pigmented lesions
Pulsed dye (PDL)	577–600	Liquid (rhodamine dye)	Hemoglobin	Superficial vascular lesions (port wine stains, telangiectasias)
Nd: YAG	1064	Crystal	Hemoglobin, melanin	Deep vascular lesions, pigmented lesions, pigmented hair
Ruby	694	Crystal	Melanin	Pigmented lesions (lentigines, nevus of Ota, tattoos), pigmented hair
Alexandrite	755	Crystal	Melanin	Pigmented lesions, removal of pigmented hair, tattoos
Diode	800–810	Semiconductor	Melanin	Pigmented lesions, removal of pigmented hair
Erbium: glass[a]	1540	Crystal	Water	Skin resurfacing
Thulium[a]	1927	Crystal	Water	Skin resurfacing
Erbium: YAG[b]	2940	Crystal	Water	Skin resurfacing
CO_2[b,c]	10600	Gas	Water	Skin resurfacing

[a] Nonablative.
[b] Ablative.
[c] May be fractional or nonfractional.

4. Induces temporary catagen phase and persistent hair loss with miniaturization and fibrosis.

5. Thermal relaxation time in mid-dermis is 20–100 ms for hair follicle melanin. Utilizes the principle of extended thermolysis so a long pulse width generally in the range of 3 ms is required.

6. Requires multiple treatment sessions at 2–4-month intervals.

7. Hair appears to "grow" as it is expelled. Extrusion takes 1–2 weeks.

8. May see perifollicular erythema for 2 days and erythema for up to 1 week.

9. Diode (800 nm) and Nd: YAG (1064 nm) are useful lasers. The latter laser is especially useful for patients with dark hair and medium dark skin as epidermal melanin is poorly absorbed at this wavelength, whereas the former laser has the highest efficacy for hair reduction in light skin patients. The alexandrite 755 laser is also useful for light skin, and the IPL (intense pulse light) device is useful for light hair in light skin patients.

> Laser hair removal works best on patients with light skin and dark hair, and worst on patients with dark skin and light hair.

10. Side effects.

    a. Postinflammatory hypo- and hyperpigmentation (hydroquinone can be useful for postinflammatory hyperpigmentation). Sun avoidance recommended before and after treatment. A test area should be considered.

    b. Leukotrichia.

    c. Paradoxical hypertrichosis – may be due to conversion of vellus hairs to terminal hairs, especially in dark skin types.

B. Tattoos[6]

1. Tattoo pigment is exogenously placed chromophore. This is a very small target and requires a very short pulse duration. This is achieved with Q-switching that allows high-energy short pulse durations in the nanosecond range (e.g., 755 QS alexandrite). The 755 picosecond alexandrite is a mode-locking laser (rather than a Q-switched laser) that produces extremely effective picosecond laser pulses.

2. Fragmentation of tattoo particles occurs by two mechanisms: (1) selective photothermolysis – laser energy converted to heat causing fragmentation of large particles and (2) photoacoustic vibration – oscillation of tattoo particles facilitates fragmentation. A localized laser heating causes thermoelastic expansion and acoustic shock waves causing disruption of pigment; there is subsequent phagocytosis and clearing. This effect is thermomechanical.

3. Pigment color determines which laser to select for best results. However, tattoo color (Table 18.4) may be produced by combination of pigments not easily seen. In general, shorter wavelengths are used for lighter colors and longer wavelengths are used for darker colors.

4. Black pigment responds best to laser treatment.

5. Homemade tattoos are one color and easiest to treat if superficial and pigment at same level but may be difficult to treat if pigment at different levels. Amateur tattoos tend to use cigarette ash, burnt wood carbon, pencil graphite, or India ink. Professional tattoos are harder to remove because the pigment is place deeper and more colors are used.

6. Requires several treatment sessions.

7. Complications.

    a. Scarring.

    b. Local allergic reaction – most common with red cinnabar (mercuric sulfide) tattoo.

    c. Immediate pigment darkening (paradoxical darkening).

TABLE 18.4

Laser Choice by Tattoo Color

Tattoo Color	Tattoo Source	QS Ruby (694 nm)	QS Alexandrite (755 nm)	QS Nd: YAG (532 nm)	QS Nd: YAG (1064 nm)
Black/dark brown	Carbon, India ink, iron oxide, gun powder	X	X		X
Blue	Cobalt	X	X		X
Green	Chromium oxide	X	X		
Red	Cinnabar, sienna			X	
Yellow	Cadmium			X	
Light brown	Ochre			X	
Violet	Manganese violet			X	
White	Titanium dioxide			X	

     i.   Most common in flesh, yellow, brown, or white colors.

    ii.   Rust color turns black due to reduction of ferric oxide (Fe_2O_3) to ferrous oxide (FeO). This can happen with red lip liner.

   iii.   White turns black or blue due to reduction of titanium (Ti^{4+} to Ti^{3+}).

   iv.   Combustion is possible during laser heating of a gunpowder tattoo.

C.   Pigmented lesions

   1.   Melanin is the target chromophore. Melanin has a wide absorption spectrum.

   2.   Longer wavelengths are less efficient but useful for deeper pigment. Shorter wavelengths are more effective for superficial epidermal pigmented lesions, whereas longer wavelengths are more effective for dermal pigmentation.

   3.   Lasers are useful for pigmented epidermal lesions, e.g., solar lentigos, lentigines, achrocordons, small seborrheic keratosis, and for some mixed epidermal/dermal lesions such as nevus of Ota, nevus of Ito. For melasma and postinflammatory hyperpigmentation, improvement is unpredictable but usually poor.

   4.   Three lasers to consider include the following.

      a.   Q-switched ruby (694 nm).

      b.   Q-switched alexandrite with or without the picosecond feature (755 nm). The small melanin in nevus of Ota is similar to tattoo pigment and may respond best to the picosecond setting.

      c.   Q-switched Nd: YAG with or without the picosecond feature (532 nm and 1064 nm).

   5.   Complications

      a.   Hyperpigmentation especially if patient on amiodarone or minocycline.

D.   Vascular lesions

   1.   Chromophore is oxyhemoglobin and hemoglobin.

   2.   Pulsed dye laser at 585 nm or 595 nm. Best for postsurgical erythema, hemangiomas, and telangiectasias. Potassium titanyl phosphate (KTP) (532 nm) useful for small angiomas, small linear or spider telangiectasias. Nd: YAG (1064 nm) can also be used.

   3.   Pulse stacking increases efficiency but may lead to skin whitening or blister formation.

   4.   Larger blood vessel targets may need pulse durations longer than the thermal relaxation time so that heat is conducted to the blood vessel walls. The heated vessel walls collapse and thus close. This effect is known as extended thermolysis.

   5.   Shorter pulse width is more effective but increases risk of purpura.

   6.   For large areas cold compresses after treatment help reduce immediate swelling and redness.

7. Total block sunscreens recommended for 1 month after treatment.
8. Problems/complications.
   a. Purpura that fades in 5–7 days.
   b. Crusting with secondary infection.
E. Skin resurfacing[5]
   1. Water is the target chromophore.
   2. Treated with ablative and nonablative lasers.
   3. Results in skin that is better hydrated, has renewed elastic properties, contains less wrinkles, and appears rejuvenated.
   4. Nonfractional (continuous wave) (Figure 18.2).
      a. Totally ablative.
         i. Effective for wrinkles and superficial pigmented lesions; these are removed in a nonspecific manner. Also used for cutting.
         ii. Uses carbon dioxide laser (10600 nm), erbium: YAG (2940 nm).
            a) Erbium: YAG has higher water absorption coefficient leading to more superficial ablation and less scatter.
            b) Carbon dioxide laser is pulsed rather than continuous mode so less tissue damage.
         iii. Water-containing tissue is vaporized.

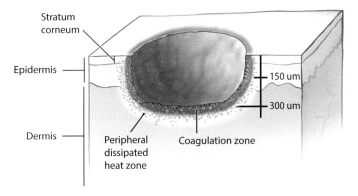

Nonfractional ablative laser wound

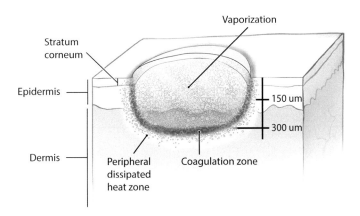

Nonfractional nonablative laser wound

FIGURE 18.2 Wounds created by (top) nonfractional ablative and (bottom) nonfractional nonablative lasers.

iv. Surrounding zone of thermal damage (coagulation zone).

v. Longer recovery time and greater risk of complications compared to nonablative lasers (see below).

vi. Ablation depth confined to epidermis and papillary dermis. Deeper ablation increases with number of passes.

vii. Tissue destruction results in stimulation of fibroblasts that produce neocollagenesis, collagen remodeling, and neovascularization followed by contraction and reepithelization.

viii. Antiviral prophylaxis suggested beginning 24 hours prior to the beginning of procedure.

ix. Contraindications: oral isotretinoin 6–12 months preceding treatment, active viral or bacterial infections, history of keloids, connective tissue disease.

x. Complications: scarring, secondary wound infection (herpes simplex, bacterial, candida), postinflammatory hyper or delayed hypopigmentation, persistent erythema.

b. Nonablative – Useful for mild wrinkle reduction.

i. Penetrates to papillary dermis, but spares much of the epidermis.

ii. Gently heats the dermis in bulk.

iii. Produces a mild collagen remodeling process.

iv. Useful lasers – Q-switched Nd: YAG (1064 nm) laser.

v. Little to no recovery time, but less dramatic results than seen with ablative laser treatments.

5. Fractional resurfacing – only a fraction of the skin surface is treated (Figure 18.3).

a. Fractional nonablative.

i. Produces columns of thermal injury (via "fractional photothermolysis") with intervening nondamaged epidermis and dermis. These columns, referred to as microthermal zones (MTZs), stamp a grid-like pattern on the skin surface that appears as tiny dots, or pixels. The diameter of each MTZ is about 100 μm and the depth of penetration is 300 μm–1.5 mm (1500 μm). The columns of injury extend deeper than ablative laser.

ii. Coagulates tissue in the MTZ's, but leaves stratum corneum intact.

iii. Uses wavelengths in the mid-infrared zone such as fractional diode (1410 nm), fractional Nd: YAG (1440 nm), Er: glass (1540 nm), fractional thulium (1927 nm), and thulium: alexandrite (1940 nm).

iv. Less downtime (3–7 days) compared to fractional ablative laser resurfacing (6–10 days).

v. May require multiple treatments.

vi. Complications: hyperpigmentation, especially in dark skin phototypes.

b. Fractional ablative.

i. Good for acne scars, skin tightening, fine wrinkle reduction.

ii. Requires one to three treatments.

iii. Works well on facial and nonfacial skin.

iv. Produces columns of microthermal injury zones. This results in microscopic necrotic debris that is vaporized in the MTZs and extrudes between 3 and 7 days followed by wound healing. There is immediate skin tightening due to collagen contraction and further skin tightening with contraction of granulation tissue within the columns (Figure 18.4).

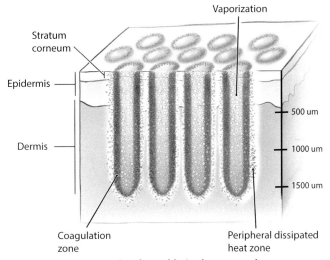

Fractional nonablative laser wound

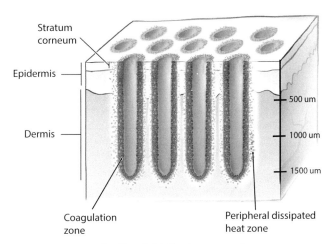

Fractional ablative laser wound

FIGURE 18.3 Wounds created by (top) fractional nonablative and (bottom) fractional ablative lasers.

     v. Complications: herpes simplex infection, bacterial infection, transient milia, posttreatment erythema.

VII. Laser Safety

    A. Eye injury is one of the most serious risks of surgical lasers (see Table 18.5). In general, mid- and far-infrared lasers damage the cornea and sclera, whereas visible and near infrared lasers can damage the uvea, iris, and retina

    B. Wavelength-specific goggles must be worn by the patient and everyone in the treatment room to provide protection against specific wavelengths of laser light

    C. The treatment room door is closed during treatment. A laser warning sign is posted outside the treatment room. No hanging mirrors are in the treatment room

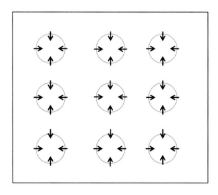

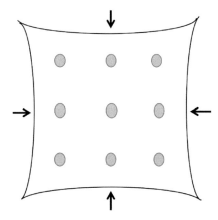

FIGURE 18.4   Top: ablative fractional injury wounds that are very small and in a grid formation. As these wounds heal, contraction occurs (arrows) and results in skin tightening (bottom).

    D. Fire is possible with laser use. A fire extinguisher should be readily available

    E. Laser key should not be left in laser when not in use

VIII. Unusual Complications

    A. Transfer of viruses by laser plume to personnel. The plume contains aerosolized tissue that can be eliminated by use of a smoke evacuator. It is recommended that a N95 mask is worn by all personnel

    B. Cavitation – a photomechanical effect of sudden tissue heating that produces a stress/shock/acoustic wave when water in skin is vaporized. Steam bubbles expand and collapse causing tissue damage and subsequent tissue shredding

During laser use, it is extremely important that the patient's eyes are covered and that goggles are worn by every other person in the room.

TABLE 18.5

Laser Light Induced Eye Injury

Type of Light	Laser Type	Wavelength	Ocular Target	Eye Effect
Visible	Ruby, PDL	400–700 nm	Retina	Blindness
Infrared A	Nd: YAG, CO_2 Erbium: glass	760–1400 nm	Retina	Blindness
Infrared B	CO_2, Erbium: glass	>1400 nm	Cornea (water)	Corneal burn

Conclusion

Lasers are highly specific and powerful light sources that have the ability to selectively destroy targets in the skin when the right laser is used at appropriate settings. They have a variety of dermatologic applications including destruction of vascular and pigmented lesions, hair removal, and skin rejuvenation. With the continued development of new lasers, their use continues to expand in both medical and cosmetic dermatology.

REFERENCES

1. Hruza G, Avram MM. Lasers and lights. In: Procedures in Cosmetic Dermatology, 3rd Edition. Elsevier, 2013.
2. Bolognia JL, Jorizzo JL, Schaffer JV. Dermatology, 3rd Edition. Elsevier, New York, NY, 2012.
3. Mann MW, Berk DR, Popkin DL, Bayliss SJ. Handbook of Dermatology: A Practical Manual. Blackwell Publishing, Chichester, West Sussex, UK, 2009.
4. Kaminer MS, Arndt KA, Dover JS, Rohrer TE. Atlas of Cosmetic Surgery, 2nd Edition. Saunders, Philadelphia, 2008.
5. Small R, Hoang D. A Practical Guide to Laser Procedures. Wolters Kluwer, Philadelphia, 2016.
6. Mariwalla K, Leffell DJ. Primer in dermatologic surgery. In: American Society for Dermatologic Surgery, 2nd Edition. Rolling Meadows, IL, 2011; pp. 115–128.

19

Sclerotherapy and Endovenous Ablation

Mitchel P. Goldman

Introduction

It has been estimated that between 10% and 20% of adults in United States and Western Europe have varicose (large dilated) leg veins and up to 50% of women by age 50 will have telangiectatic (very small dilated) leg veins. While most patients who present for treatment do so for cosmetic reasons, up to 50% of patients with varicose veins will develop symptoms or adverse sequellae, including superficial thrombophlebitis and leg ulceration. The difference between varicose, reticular, and telangiectatic leg veins is one of size. By convention, a tortuous vein greater than 4–5 mm in diameter is referred to as varicose, a vein between 1 and 4 mm in diameter is referred to as reticular, and a vein less than 1 mm in diameter is referred to as telangiectatic.[1] Telangiectatic vessels can be further subcategorized as linear, arborizing, or spider (Figure 19.1).

The most common misconception among treating physicians is that these unwanted dilated veins can be treated independently from one another. While a telangiectasia can be treated without thought to its cause (always a feeding incompetent reticular vein), independent treatment will result in a high risk of pigmentation and telangiectatic matting, as well as requiring multiple treatments. When one realizes that ALL superficial veins are interconnected and not separate entities (since the blood that flows through them must come from somewhere), one can treat these veins in one procedure with little, if any, adverse effects.

    I. Pathophysiology

        A. The most common predisposing factors for the development of "unwanted" leg veins are the following

            1. Family history.

            2. Any activity or condition that increases abdominal pressure and impedes the flow of venous blood back to the heart may put strain on the veins causing them to dilate.

    (a)   (b)   (c)

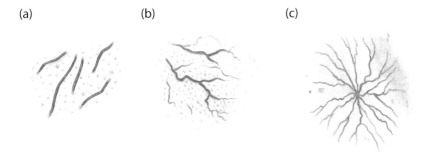

FIGURE 19.1 Types of telangiectasias. (A) Linear, (B) Arborizing, and (C) Spider. (Reproduced with permission from Bennett RG. *Fundamentals of Cutaneous Surgery.* C.V. Mosby, St. Louis, 1988.)

     a. Standing for long periods of time.

     b. Lack of exercise.

     c. Obesity.

     d. Constipation.

     e. Wearing high-heel shoes (which requires one to walk using the buttock muscles and not the calf or foot muscles).

     f. Wearing tight undergarments or pants (producing a tourniquet effect on the proximal superficial veins).

3. The use of estrogen and/or progesterone hormone supplementation for birth control or for postmenopausal symptoms also causes a dilatation of the vein wall.

4. Localized trauma (e.g., being hit with a tennis ball or other object) may initiate angiogenesis with the eruption of a telangiectasia. Also, localized trauma may damage perforating veins leading to an increase in blood flow from the deep to superficial circulations.

5. Photodamage from the sun or other forms of radiation are also associated with an increase in telangiectasia through degradation of the supporting elastic and collagen network surrounding blood vessels.

6. Pregnancy puts strain on veins by increasing blood volume, increasing estrogen and progesterone, and impeding blood flow through compression of the pelvic venous system.

7. Age. Varicose, reticular, and/or telangiectatic veins appear in 1/3 of patients before age 25 and increase in incidence with age. By age 70, 70% of individuals have visible cutaneous leg veins.

II. Laboratory Findings and Diagnosis

A. Irrespective of the underlying cause of venous dilatation, the source of backflow, whether incompetent perforating veins, feeding reticular veins, or an incompetent saphenofemoral junction (SFJ), must be treated first

B. Duplex ultrasound examination takes 2–5 minutes and determines if the great saphenous vein (GSV) is abnormal with a reversal of blood flow

    1. The duplex ultrasound is much easier to master than the stethoscope and must be used by any physician who treats unwanted dilated leg veins. A complete discussion on the relative merits of this technique is found elsewhere.[1]

III. Treatment

A. Sclerotherapy is usually done by injecting a sclerosing solution into a vein to produce a "controlled" thrombophlebotic reaction. Therefore, the main principle is to produce the least amount of collateral damage (i.e., inflammation). The commonly used sclerosing agents are shown in Table 19.1

    1. Minimizing inflammation by injecting the vessel with the minimally effective sclerosing concentration will avoid the risk of initiating new telangiectasias from forming around the treated area edges.

    2. Graduated compression immediately after sclerotherapy will minimize resulting inflammation by decreasing thrombus formation.

B. Sclerotherapy should progress from the largest to smallest vessels. This will allow cannulation and infusion of the sclerosing solution to occur most easily

> Sclerotherapy should progress from the largest vessels to the smallest vessels.

    1. Often, with injection of larger reticular veins first, solution is seen entering telangiectasias which they feed into, thus obviating the need to cannulate the distal smaller telangiectasias.

TABLE 19.1

Comparison of Sclerosing Agents for Various Size Veins

	Endothelial Cell Damage/Result	**Telangiectatic Veins** **<1 mm**	**Reticular Veins** **1–4 mm**	**Varicose Veins** **4–10 mm**
HS[a] 11.7%	Osmotic dehydration/destruction fibrin, thrombosis	X		
Glycerin (72%)	Irritation/endosclerosis	X		
STS[b] Foam 0.25%	Cell surface lipids/desquamation	X		
STS Foam 0.25%–0.5%	Cell surface lipids/desquamation		X	
STS Foam 1%–3%	Cell surface lipids/desquamation			X
POL[c] Foam 0.5%	Cell surface lipids/desquamation	X		
POL Foam 0.5%–1%	Cell surface lipids/desquamation		X	
POL 2%–5%,	Cell surface lipids/desquamation			X

[a] Hypertonic saline.

[b] Sodium tetradecyl sulfate.

[c] Polidocanol.

C. The quantity of sclerosing solution to be injected should be enough to fill the vessel and displace intravascular blood
   1. When you stop seeing the solution flowing, you should stop the injection as this means that the solution is flowing into the deeper venous system.

D. The entire venous system of each leg is treated at one time to avoid leaving areas of refluxing blood flow, which may cause recanalization of the treated vessel, or extravasation of red blood cells from the damaged vessel that leads to hyperpigmentation

E. Foamed sclerosing solutions are recommended for all veins greater than 1 mm in diameter
   1. Can only be done with a detergent sclerosing solution such as sodium tetradecyl sulfate ([STS] Sotradecol) or polidocanol ([POL] Asclera).
   2. Mix 1 mL of solution with 4 mL of air.
   3. Foaming a sclerosing solution increases its effective sclerosing power by two while decreasing its adverse effect profile by four since the solution is diluted four-fold by air.

F. Patients should be examined 2 weeks after injection so that any area of thrombosis (representing trapped blood and always called a "coagulum" to the patient) can be evacuated early through a 22-gauge needle
   1. Evacuation of the coagulum will minimize the appearance of hyperpigmentation and speed resorption of the destroyed blood vessel.

G. The treated area should not be retreated sooner than 6–8 weeks after injection to allow for resolution of inflammation between treatments

H. The patient is instructed to walk immediately after the injection session to help compress the superficial and perforating veins and prevent deep vein thrombosis
   1. Calf muscle movement produces a rapid blood flow in the deep venous system that dilutes out any sclerosant that may have migrated to this area.

I. Following injection of all varicose, reticular, or telangiectatic veins, the treated veins are compressed to minimize significant thrombosis[2–5]
   1. Graduated compression eliminates a thrombophlebitic reaction and substitutes a "sclerophlebitis" with the production of a firm fibrous cord.

After a sclerotherapy session, leg compression with graduated compression stockings is key to increase success and minimizing complications.

2. Compression, if adequate, may result in direct apposition of the treated vein walls to produce a more effective fibrosis.

3. Compressing the treated vessel will decrease the extent of thrombus formation that inevitably occurs with the use of all sclerosing solutions, thus decreasing the risk for recanalization of the treated vessel.

    a. A decrease in the extent of thrombus formation may also decrease the incidence of postsclerotherapy pigmentation.

    b. The limitation of thrombosis and phlebitic reactions may prevent the appearance of angiogenesis/telangiectatic matting.

4. The function of the calf muscle pump is improved by the physiologic effect of a graduated compression stocking.

    a. By externally supporting untreated large veins, compression stockings will narrow vein diameter, restoring competency to its valvular function, which decreases retrograde blood flow.

    b. External pressure will also retard the reflux of blood from incompetent perforating veins into the superficial veins.

5. Graduated compression stockings have been shown to minimize the development of postsclerotherapy hyperpigmentation, cutaneous necrosis, and telangiectatic matting even for veins less than 1 mm in diameter.

J. Microsclerotherapy

1. A 2-power loupe for magnification is helpful to aid visualization.

2. A 30-gauge needle is sufficient (Figure 19.2).

3. For vessels less than 1 mm in diameter, I have found that a 72% glycerin solution mixed 2:1 with 1% lidocaine with epinephrine is best.[6]

    a. With this sclerosing solution, there is virtually no risk of ulceration, pigmentation, and telangiectatic matting.

    b. Resolution of the veins appears better than with a detergent solution.

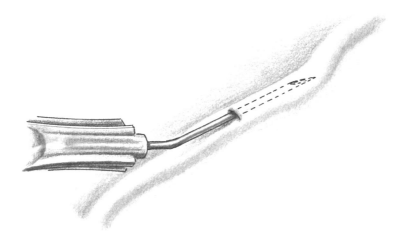

FIGURE 19.2 Telangiectasia being injected with sclerosing agent using a 30-gauge needle slightly bent with the bevel up. (Reproduced with permission from Bennett RG, *Fundamentals of Cutaneous Surgery*. C.V. Mosby, St. Louis, 1988.)

IV. Course and Prognosis

A. Unfortunately, as with any therapeutic technique, sclerotherapy carries with it a number of potential adverse sequelae and complications. Fortunately, these complications are quite rare

  1. Fairly common adverse sequelae include the following.

     a. Temporary perivascular cutaneous hyperpigmentation.

     b. Temporary flare of new perivascular telangiectasias.

  2. Relatively rare complications include the following.

     a. Localized cutaneous necrosis. Hypertonic saline carries highest risk.

     b. Thrombophlebitis of the injected vessel.

     c. Arterial injection with resultant distal necrosis. See immediate skin blanching and patient complains of intense burning pain.

     d. Pulmonary emboli.

     e. Anaphylaxis (especially with sodium morrhuate).

V. Endovenous Albation

A. Used when reflux detected in GSV

B. Devices used

  1. Radiofrequency.

     a. Used with tumescent anesthesia.

     b. Threaded into varicose veins distally through ultrasonic guidance.

     c. As catheter is withdrawn, radiofrequency heat is applied to the vein wall, which causes collagen in the vein wall to shrink.

  2. Endovenous laser targeting hemoglobin (810 nm, 940 nm, 980 nm).

     a. Used with tumescent anesthesia.

     b. Laser energy absorbed by hemoglobin and red blood cells, which heats endothelial cells causing vein walls to collapse and fibrose.

     c. Outcome affected by amount of red blood cells in the vein and the rate of pullback.

  3. Endovenous laser targeting tissue water (1320 nm, 1450 nm).

     a. Heats water around collagen and vein walls resulting in collagen damage and fibrosis.

     b. Less heat, less pain, and less bruising compared to laser devices targeting water molecule.

     c. Device has automatic pullback.

Conclusion

Sclerotherapy is a fast, relatively easy method to obliterate unsightly telangiectasias and varicose veins. Nevertheless, this technique requires careful patient choice, sclerosing agent selection, and experience.

REFERENCES

1. Goldman MP, Guex JJ, Weiss RA, editors. Sclerotherapy Treatment of Varicose and Telangiectatic Leg Veins: Diagnosis and Treatment. 6th Edition. Elsevier, London, 2016.
2. Goldman MP. How to Utilize Compression after Sclerotherapy. Dermatol Surg 2002; 28: 860–862.

3. Goldman MP. Treatment of Varicose and Telangiectatic Leg Veins: Double Blind Prospective Comparative Trial between Aethoxysklerol and Sotradecol. Dermatol Surg 2002; 28: 52–55.
4. Barrett JM, Allen B, Ockelford A, Goldman MD. Microfoam Ultrasound Guided Sclerotherapy of Varicose Veins in 100 Legs. Dermatol Surg 2004; 30: 6–12.
5. Weiss RA, Sadick NS, Goldman MP, Weiss MA. Post-Sclerotherapy Compression and Its Effects on Clinical Outcome. Dermatol Surg 1999; 25: 105–108.
6. Leach B, Goldman MP. Comparative Trial between Sodium Tetradecyl Sulfate and Glycerin in the Treatment of Telangiectatic Leg Veins. Dermatol Surg 2003; 29: 612–625.

20

Tumescent Liposuction

William P. Coleman III and Kyle Coleman

Introduction

Liposuction is performed through a hollow cannula attached to a suction machine and is used to manually remove adipose tissue to improve body contours. Modern liposuction can trace its roots to the European innovations in the late 1970s.[1] In 1982–1983, liposuction was introduced to the United States through numerous specialty society meetings. Included among these was dermatology, which would become an integral part of the future developments in body contouring.

In the beginning, liposuction was primarily performed under general anesthesia; however, under general, the procedure was initially fraught with complications such as hematomas, seromas, hemodilution, infections, and death. Dermatologists pioneered the use of local anesthesia for liposuction, but were limited by the side effects associated with large volumes of lidocaine. In 1987, a dermatologist, Dr. Jeffrey Klein, published his work on "tumescent anesthesia", a novel technique that uses large volumes of very dilute lidocaine to produce profound anesthesia in the skin and subcutaneous space.[2] This tumescent technique allowed large volume liposuction to be efficiently and more safely performed in an outpatient office setting rather than in an operating room. Over the next decade, hundreds of thousands of liposuction procedures were performed in this manner. Data from these cases showed that the tumescent technique had vastly superior safety compared to liposuction under general anesthesia in an operating room. Today tumescent liposuction is the gold standard in body contouring.[3,4]

> Tumescent liposuction was a major advance for liposuction, in that, liposuction could be performed much more safely than under general anesthesia.

  I. Consultation

    A. Medical history

       1. Blood pressure.

       2. Weight/height.

       3. Past medical/surgical history.

       4. Current medications.

       5. Medication allergies.

       6. Tobacco/alcohol history.

    B. Contraindications

       1. Medically prescribed blood thinners.

       2. Obesity.

       3. Uncontrolled diabetes, hypertension.

       4. Bleeding disorders.

       5. Body dysmorphic disorders.

    C. Potential candidates

       1. Realistic expectations for improvement. Will not improve cellulite or flabby skin. Liposuction does not target the cause of cellulite or increase skin tone.

       2. Not a weight loss surgery; liposuction improves body contours.

       3. Physical examination for scarring/hernias/prior liposuction.

       4. Areas amenable to liposuction (Figure 20.1).

    D. Commitment

       1. Willingness to complete postoperative compression.

       2. Willingness to maintain weight after liposuction.

       3. Understanding of the process; liposuction is not an overnight fix.

II. Preoperative Preparation

    A. Laboratory

       1. Complete blood count (CBC).

       2. Comprehensive metabolic profile.

       3. Protime (PT) and partial thromboplastin time (PTT).

       4. Pregnancy testing.

    B. Medications. Several medications are typically used intraoperatively

       1. Antibiotics, generally broad spectrum, such as cephalosporins.

       2. Anxiolytics, generally benzodiazepines, for day of surgery.

       3. Pain control, possible narcotics. Liposuction is generally a well-tolerated procedure requiring minimal postoperative pain medications.

    C. Consent for procedure should include

       1. Areas to be treated.

       2. Possible liposuction side effects: asymmetry, irregular contours, skin laxity, nerve injury, pain, swelling, bruising.

       3. Possible side effects related to all surgery: blood clots, infection, hospitalization, and death.

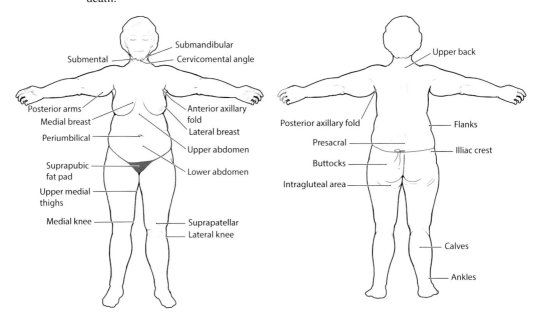

FIGURE 20.1 Locations amenable to liposuction. Left: anterior view, Right: posterior view. Women typically store the most fat in the hips. Men store the fibrous fat in the flanks and breast and most fat in the flanks.

D. Instructions

   1. Patients will require a driver and someone to stay with them at home for 24 hours after surgery.

   2. Patients will have drainage of the anesthetic fluid for up to 48 hours from the skin incisions.

   3. Patients will wear postoperative compression garments for 2–12 weeks determined by the area treated and patient physical characteristics.

   4. Patients will follow up with the physician at a predetermined schedule.

   5. Patients understand the procedure itself, the expected results, and the importance of following pre- and postoperative protocols.

III. Tumescent Anesthesia

A. The following agents are combined to formulate the tumescent anesthetic solution[3]

   1. Generally prepared in 500 mL to 1 L of normal saline.

   2. Lidocaine 0.05%–0.1%.

   3. 1:1,000,000–1:2,000,000 epinephrine.

   4. 10 mEq of sodium bicarbonate.

FORMULA FOR 0.05% LIDOCAINE TUMESCENT SOLUTION

- 50 cc 1% plain lidocaine (500 mg)
- 1 cc 1:1000 epinephrine (1 mg)
- 10 mEq sodium bicarbonate (8.4% $NaHCO_3$ solution)
- 1 liter normal saline (0.9% NaCl solution)

B. Administration

   1. The prepared tumescent anesthetic solution is infiltrated slowly and subcutaneously using a peristaltic pump. This should be done by a physician or experienced staff member under onsite supervision.

   2. Infiltration is performed via a 16-gauge to 18-gauge specially designed cannula (Figure 20.2A).

   3. Fluid is infiltrated into the subcutaneous space until appropriate skin turgor and blanching occurs.

C. Advantages of tumescent liposuction

   1. Creation of enlarged tissue planes to facilitate cannula insertion.

   2. Creates tissue firmness (turgor) that helps the physician to manually sense the location and the effectiveness of the cannula as it removes fat.

   3. Less trauma to surrounding tissue (protects muscle, nerve, blood vessels).

   4. Minimal bruising/pain.

D. Advantages of tumescent liposuction without general anesthesia

   1. Patients may eat prior to surgery thus reducing nausea and avoiding hypoglycemia. There is no need for the patient to fast or be *nil per os* (NPO) before the procedure.

   2. Lasting anesthesia of the areas infiltrated (3–24 hours).

   3. Intraoperative patient mobility – as the patient is awake and able to move during the procedure, $360°$ contouring is possible.

   4. Little likelihood of complications such as infection, fluid shift problems, or deep vein thrombosis.

   5. No reported deaths with tumescent anesthesia without general anesthesia in the United States.[5]

E. Potential side effects

   1. Temporary edema in untreated sites.

   2. Tachycardia.

   3. Lidocaine toxicity. Although reports have shown dosages of up to 55 mg/kg of tumescent anesthesia are safe in conjunction with liposuction, 45 mg/kg would give

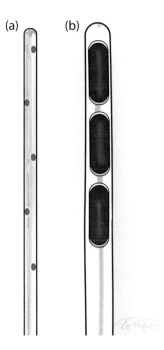

FIGURE 20.2   (A) Tumescent anesthetic infiltration cannula. Note blunt tip with multiple small ports. These extend 360°
around for even fluid distribution and (B) Liposuction cannula. Note blunt tip and large ports.

an extra margin of safety. Patients must avoid medications that potentially inhibit
lidocaine metabolism by the liver. Specifically, lidocaine is metabolized by the
hepatic microsomal enzyme cytochrome P450 3A4 (CYP3A4). Other drugs that
are metabolized by CYP3A4 will interfere with lidocaine metabolism and should
be discontinued prior to liposuction.[3]

IV. Liposuction Procedure

  A.   Instrumentation

    1.   Cannulas – differing size diameters and shapes. Generally, blunt with multiple ports
through which adipose tissue is extracted (Figure 20.2B).

    2.   Tubing – sterile, one-time use connects the cannula to the suction machine.
Aspiration has been found to be directly proportional to the suction tubing diameter
and inversely proportional to the suction tubing length.[6]

    3.   Suction – continuous negative pressure of 20–30 mmHg.

  B.   Technique

    1.   Photographs: preoperative photographs are taken of the areas to be treated.
Careful attention is paid to body posture/positioning and lighting for reproducible
photographs.

    2.   Markings: patients are marked standing with a surgical marker in the areas to be suc-
tioned prior to administration of tumescent fluid. The fluid infiltration will later distort
the areas to be treated.

    3.   Incisions: small incisions of 2–4 mm are made with a scalpel blade (15c, 15, or 11) or
skin punch. Generally, these incision wounds are left unsutured after the liposuction
procedure to allow drainage of tumescent anesthetic.

    4.   Tunneling: cannulas are inserted subcutaneously to create tunnels in the adipose layer
in differing depths.

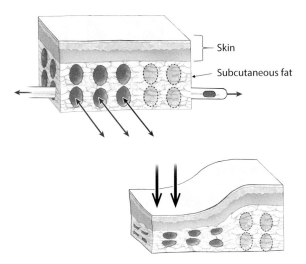
Skin

Subcutaneous fat

FIGURE 20.3 Tissue tunneling (Top). Fat removed with liposuction cannula in multiple planes from multiple directions. Thus, cross-tunnels are created. (Bottom) Collapse of adipose tissue after fat extraction.

5. Cross-tunneling: multiple tunnels are created from several directions to create consistent tissue contraction as occurs in a sponge (Figure 20.3).

6. End point: consistent flaccidity throughout the treated area and even subcutaneous layer thickness.

V. Postoperative Care

A. Day of surgery

1. Ambulation/normal diet encouraged.

2. Increased oral intake of water encouraged.

3. Recommend resting at home with adult supervision.

B. Incision wounds

1. Absorbent padding placed over wounds for the drainage of tumescent anesthetic fluid.

2. Once drainage has stopped, wound care with white petrolatum (Vaseline®) applied to wounds to encourage healing.

3. Resultant scars may need postoperative treatment for hyperpigmentation in darker skinned individuals, as with all scars.

4. No submersion in water until wounds are fully healed; however, patients may shower one day after surgery.

C. Garments

1. Compressive garments are worn to decrease swelling in the areas treated in order to maximize tissue collapse and contraction.

2. Garments are worn for 24 hours for the first 2 weeks after surgery. Gradually, the garments become less restrictive and are worn less often.

3. Help decrease bruising and potential for seroma/hematoma formation.

D. Follow-up

1. Patients generally are seen on the day after surgery, 1–2 weeks later, then quarterly.

2. Patients are reminded that garments are an essential part of the procedure.

3. Patients are to maintain a healthy diet and control their weight.

4. Light exercise is allowed starting on the second day after surgery. Exercise to be increased as tolerated. Patients are encouraged to exercise regularly.

5. Results from liposuction take time. Like a scar, tissue remodeling and collagen deposition take place over a 12-month period with the majority of the contraction taking place over the first 3–6 months. Patients are generally happy with results at 6–12 weeks after surgery but results will continue to improve over time.

6. Postoperative photographs are taken as early as 6 weeks to as late as 1 year.

VI. Recent Innovations

A. The following devices have been used to assist with liposuction and more efficaciously remove fat. Usually, these devices are incorporated into the liposuction cannula

1. Lasers – provide coagulation of small blood vessels, rupture of fat cells, and coagulation of collagen. May promote skin tightening; however, there is currently no conclusive evidence for any benefit at this time.[6]

2. Ultrasound – provides vibration amplification of sound energy to generate heat for fat cell disruption and tissue tightening. There is no proven advantage to using this method.[6]

3. Radiofrequency – provides heating of deep fat tissue. May result in improved skin tightening.[6]

4. Water assisted – provides pulsating water jets of tumescent solution from a dual purpose cannula that simultaneously suctions fat tissue and fluid. Not enough evidence at this time to support a cosmetic benefit.[6]

VII. Miscellaneous Indications for Liposuction

A. Liposuction has been recommended to remove lipomas and for axillary hyperhidrosis. Our experience is that liposuction is less than optimal for these indications

Conclusion

Tumescent liposuction is the gold standard in body contouring. The procedure is safe and effective with a high degree of patient satisfaction. Tumescent liposuction has distinct advantages over liposuction performed under general anesthesia.

REFERENCES

1. Coleman WP III. Liposuction and Anesthesia. Dermatol Surg 1987; 13: 1295–1296.
2. Klein JA. The Tumescent Technique for Liposuction Surgery. Am J Cosmetic Surg 1987; 4: 263–267.
3. Klein JA. Tumescent Technique for Local Anesthesia Improves Safety in Large-Volume Liposuction. Plast Reconstr Surg 1993; 92: 1085–1098.
4. Habbema L. Safety of Liposuction Using Exclusively Tumescent Local Anesthesia in 3,240 Consecutive Cases. Dermatol Surg 2009; 35: 1728–1735.
5. Housman TS, Lawrence N, Mellen BG et al. The Safety of Liposuction: Results of a National Survey. Dermatol Surg 2002; 28: 971–978.
6. Chia CT, Neinstein RM, Theodorou SJ. Evidence-Based Medicine: Liposuction. Plat Reconstr Surg. 2017; 139: 267e–274e.

21

Hair Transplantation

Paul McAndrews

Introduction

Hair transplantation is as much an art as it is a science. If the fundamentals of hair transplant surgery are not performed correctly, the grafts do not survive; however, if the artistic parts of the transplant are not properly applied, the doctor and patient will wish the grafts do not survive.

Dermatologists developed and popularized hair transplantation that is founded on the concept of "donor dominance".[1] This concept is predicated by knowledge that the donor hair-bearing graft that is utilized for transplantation will survive in the recipient wound and its hairs will grow at the same rate, thickness, and color as it did in the donor area, regardless of the recipient site location. Since the most common form of hair loss treated today is androgenetic alopecia, it is understandable that the most common area where hair transplantation is performed is the scalp. Good genetic hair, typically from the sides and back of the scalp, is transferred to an area of hair loss. Good genetic hair is hair that will not fall out over time and grows at the same rate and thickness as it did originally. Further, it is not susceptible to hormonal influences. However, other forms of hair loss may also be treated with hair transplantation; these areas include eyebrows, beard, and scars in hair-bearing areas (i.e., cleft lip scar).

> Hair transplantation is based on the concept of donor dominance; that is, once it vascularizes, a hair containing skin graft will continue to grow hair. In addition, gray hair when transplanted continues to grow gray.

I. Androgenetic Alopecia

    A. Most common form of hair loss

    B. The genetically susceptible hair progressively miniaturizes under the influence of dihydrotestosterone (DHT) until it cannot be seen by the naked eye

    C. Progressive process every human experiences to some degree with aging

    D. The individual genetics dictate the severity and pattern of hair loss[2]

    E. One cannot clinically detect balding until there is a 50% decrease in hair density[3]

II. Limitations of Hair Transplantations[4]

    A. Unwise to perform in patients with lichen planopilaris, discoid lupus, or other inflammatory conditions of the scalp

    B. Keloids are possible if the patient is a keloid former. Consider a few test hair transplants to see if keloids will form in the transplant or donor sites

    C. Patients on blood thinners and multiple medications may be at risk for poor graft survival

    D. Limited amount of healthy hair that can be transferred to the area of concern.[5] Hair transplant surgeons have been said to be glorified farmers; they potentially have 10 acres of land to cover, but only have 4 acres of seed (Figure 21.1)[6]

        1. Move healthy hair wisely to where it is most cosmetically important (Figure 21.2). The frontal and mid-scalp are the most essential areas to have hair.

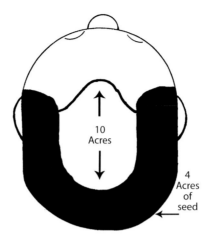

FIGURE 21.1   Only a limited number of hairs can be harvested on sides and back of scalp to completely cover the bald area on top of scalp.

      a. Frontal mid-scalp hair frames your face, follows a natural balding process, and hair in this area can be brushed backward to hide the balding vertex.

      b. The medical therapies for androgenetic alopecia work best in the vertex.

2. Unwise use of the good genetic hair can create a very unnatural look with time and further balding (Figures 21.3 and 21.4).[1,2] Vertex baldness is always progressive. With time hair loss peripheral to a vertex transplantation looks unnatural. Generally, patients younger than age 25 are not good candidates for hair transplantation because their hair loss pattern over time is not stable or predictable. Also, vertex hair transplantation is more challenging because the natural hair pattern in the vertex is difficult to recreate.

3. Use techniques that ensure the highest survival of the hair-bearing grafts.

4. Adjuvant use of medical therapies (e.g., finasteride [Propecia®, Merck, Kenilworth, New Jersey] and minoxidil [Rogaine™, Johnson & Johnson, New Brunswick, New Jersey]) can be helpful for androgenetic alopecia.

      a. Decreases the progression of androgenetic alopecia.[7]

      b. Decreases the amount of hair transplants needed over time to maintain hair density.

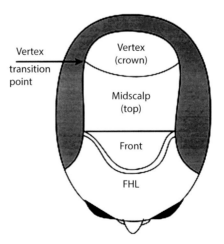

FIGURE 21.2   Potential recipient areas for hair transplants. FHL – frontal hairline.

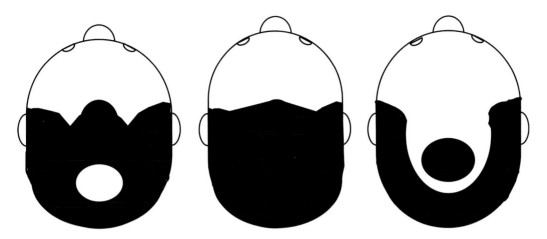

FIGURE 21.3 Hair transplantation of vertex balding. Patient has balding vertex (left) that when transplanted gives good coverage (middle) and results in the temporarily happy patient, but with time and normal balding, the transplanted vertex looks unnatural (right).

    c.   Minoxidil.
         i.   Produces larger, thicker hairs.
        ii.   Prolongs anagen phase.
      iii.   Reverses miniaturization.
      iv.   Mechanism of action unknown but some proposed ideas are enhanced follicular DNA synthesis, vasodilation, angiogenesis, and immunosuppression.
    d.   Finasteride.
         i.   Inhibits Type II 5-alpha reductase: 5-alpha reductase converts testosterone to DHT, especially on top of scalp.
        ii.   Reverses miniaturization.
      iii.   Increases hair counts.
      iv.   Decreases conversion of testosterone to DHT.
  5. Female pattern alopecia is different from that than in men. It is often more diffuse, making women poor surgical candidates. However, women with only a frontal thinning pattern can be successfully transplanted.

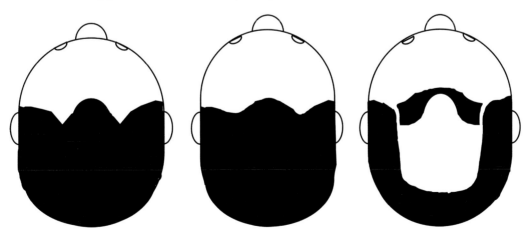

FIGURE 21.4 Hair transplantation of frontotemporal receding hairline (left) results in a temporarily happy patient (middle) but with time, normal hair loss on top of scalp results in unnatural frontal hairline (right).

III. Mechanics of Hair Transplantation

  A. "Hair Bank"

    1. Good genetic hair is unlikely to fall out during a person's lifetime.

    2. Good genetic hair available for transplantation is found around the sides and back of the scalp. There are approximately 6,250 follicular unit grafts in these areas that can be safely removed over a person's lifetime.[8]

    3. Approximately 50% of hair on the sides and back of scalp can be removed without producing noticeable baldness.[3]

  B. Donor harvesting

    1. Caution needs to be exercised not to remove hair from too high up or too low on the sides and back of the scalp since these areas may be susceptible in the future to the miniaturization process of androgenetic alopecia. Generally, the donor area is on the lateral occipital scalp from the level of the occipital protuberance to about 1 cm above the top of ears.

    2. It is best to utilize as little of the good genetic hair as possible to make the patient happy, and save the remainder for the future.

    3. Technique.

      a. Strip excision and graft dissection.

        i. A donor strip of scalp is excised in order to get the number of grafts necessary (i.e., 16 cm × 1 cm will yield 1,600 follicular unit grafts assuming there is 100 follicular units/cm^2 in the donor region). Donor strip not to exceed 30 cm × 1 cm.

> Over time, smaller and smaller hair-containing grafts have come to be used to give a more natural appearance.

        ii. The resultant donor surgical wound is then sutured (a 16 cm by 1 cm strip typically creates a 16 cm × 1 mm scar = 160 mm² of scar).

        iii. The hair-bearing strip of scalp is subdivided by sharp dissection to produce individual follicular unit grafts using the naked eye, magnifying loops, or the stereoscopic microscope. The latter gives you the best visualization that should decrease inadvertent transection of hair follicles. Each follicular unit contains one to four terminal hairs, one to two vellus hairs, sebaceous glands, and arrector pili muscles. For a natural non-hairline result, need 25–30 follicular units/cm^2; for a natural hairline result, need >40 follicular units/cm^2. Follicular unit density is calculated by the number of hairs per cm^2 divided by the number of follicular units within that cm^2.

        iv. Benefits of this technique.

          a) Less transection (since there is full visualization while dissecting the grafts as opposed to blind dissection with follicular unit extraction [FUE] technique [see below]), which equates to increased graft survival.

          b) Less surface area of total scar tissue in the donor region.

          c) Subsequent surgeries can remove prior scar (keeps the total surface area of scar to a minimum).

          d) Removes donor hair from the best genetic area.

      b. FUE by punch excision.

        i. Each individual follicular unit is removed separately with a 0.6–1.4 mm punch.

        ii. There are several different types of punches: manual, motorized, and robotic.

iii.   The donor site holes are left to heal by second intention (granulation, contraction, and re-epidermization).

iv.   The benefit is there is no linear scarring at donor site; however, there will be multiple small circular scars ($1,600 \times 1$ mm punch excisions create approximately $1,600 \times 1.2$ mm² of scar = $1,920$ mm² of surface scar tissue).

v.   The disadvantages of this technique are the following:

a)   The scalp has to be shaved before the surgery, which can be a temporary cosmetic concern.

b)   Every follicular unit graft is created by blind excision.

- This creates a situation where there is huge variability between physicians when performing the harvesting procedure.

- While using this technique, the odds of damaging hair follicles is increased as transections of some follicular units is inevitable.

c)   Each subsequent surgery adds more and more scar surface area to the donor region (subsequent surgeries do not remove scar tissue).

d)   In order to spread out the accumulating scar tissue in the donor region, many physicians tend to remove hair too high and too low in the donor regions that are genetically prone to miniaturizing with time, creating a hair transplant that becomes less visible with time.

C.   Graft storage solution

1.   There are many different storage solutions used to store the grafts during the transplant process. All these solutions contain water and electrolytes that prevent osmotic graft swelling that would occur with sterile water.

a.   Normal saline.

b.   Multiple electrolyte solution (PlasmaLyte A® [Baxter Healthcare Corporation, Deerfield, IL]).

c.   Buffered solution (HypoThermosol® [BioLife Solutions, Bothell, WA]).

2.   Consideration should be given to solutions that would minimize the trauma and maximize survival.

D.   Recipient incisions

1.   Instruments.

a.   There are numerous types of blades, needles, and "cut to fit" razor blades to create the recipient sites.

b.   The recipient site should be as small as possible to properly secure the graft without traumatizing it.

2.   Direction and angle: the angle and direction of the future graft are dictated by this initial incision which is very important in the overall naturalness of the hair transplant.

E.   Graft placement – the most common instrument utilized to place the grafts is fine tip forceps such as jewelers forceps. However, there are several implanting devices on the market. The bottoms of the grafts are generally placed to a depth of 4–6 mm

F.   Postoperative course

1.   Sutures in the recipient site are removed in 1–2 weeks.

2.   Hair shafts usually fall out (posttransplant effluvium) in 2–4 weeks (follicle is still intact). Mechanism not known.

3.   Hair starts to grow at 3–4 months. Transplanted hairs may be initially more kinky than those in donor area but return to normal texture in 6–12 months.

4.   Results seen in 1 year.

G.   Postoperative problems

1. Forehead edema – usually 2–3 days postoperatively.
2. Infection.
3. Erythema of recipient site – normal for 1 week posttransplant.
4. No hair growth in transplanted grafts.
    a. Possibly due to overhandling prior to insertion.
    b. Desiccation can interfere with graft take.
5. Cobblestone appearance of donor grafts – more common if skin punch used to provide donor grafts.
6. Sterile folliculitis due to ingrown hairs due to transplanted hair being trapped as new hairs begin to grow.

IV. Artistry of a hair transplants and hairline design. An artist creates artwork by visualization of the final product in the future as opposed to a craftsman who recreates his work by copying.

> The most important aspect of hair transplantation to produce an excellent result is choosing where to place the hair-containing grafts.

A. Anterior starting point of the frontal hairline (FHL) – be cautious not to start it too far forward (Figure 21.5) since it can eventually give you an unnatural "hair piece" look[1]

B. Lateral ending point of FHL
    1. The frontotemporal hairline should be concave in a person with significant hair loss.
    2. The concave frontotemporal hairline should ascend going anterior to posterior.
    3. The frontotemporal hairline meets the temporal/parietal hairline to create an angle; this angle is the apex of what is referred to as the frontotemporal triangle. Normally, the apex of this triangle is at the top of a vertical sagittal line that runs inferiorly to the lateral canthus (Figure 21.6).

C. Hair angle and direction of FHL
    1. Follow the angle and direction of the existing miniaturized hairs.
    2. Typically, the angle of the hair exiting the scalp becomes much more acute as one looks more anterior on the scalp.

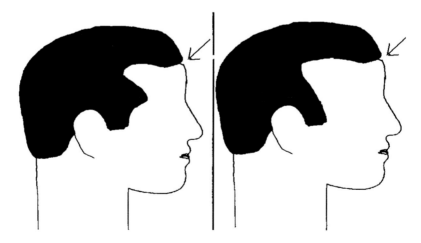

FIGURE 21.5   Placing frontal hairline too far forward (left) can create an unnatural hair piece look (right) with normal frontotemporal recession over time.

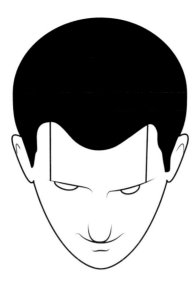

FIGURE 21.6 The apex of the frontotemporal triangle is at the top of a vertical sagittal line that runs inferiorly to the lateral canthus.

D. Irregularity of the hairline
1. Hairlines are naturally irregular.
2. A common mistake is to create a symmetric, straight FHL that looks unnatural. The human eye is drawn to straight lines rather than crooked lines.
3. The natural hairline has both large irregularities ("Widow's peak") and small irregularities (hair clusters) that need to be considered.

Conclusion

There is no perfect treatment for androgenetic alopecia, so it is imperative to inform the patient about all forms of treatment (cosmetic, medical and surgical) and then let the patient decide what is in his or her best interest. Hair transplantation when applied properly is very satisfying to the patient. However, there are times the patient should not have a hair transplant because he or she is not realistic about what can be achieved.

REFERENCES

1. Habif TP. Clinical Dermatology: A Color Guide to Diagnosis and Therapy. 3rd Edition. Mosby Year Book Inc., St Louis, MO, 1996; p. 744.
2. Hamilton JB. Patterned Loss of Hair in Men; Types and Incidence. Ann NY Acad Sci 1951; 53(3): 708–728.
3. Limmer BL. The Density Issue in Hair Transplantation. Dermatol Surg 1997; 23(9): 747–750.
4. McAndrews PJ. Hair loss and hair transplantation. In: Comprehensive Aesthetic Rejuvenation: A Regional Approach (Series in Cosmetic and Laser Therapy). 1st Edition (Kim J, Lask GP, Nelson A, editors). CRC Press, Boca Raton, 2012; 121–130.
5. McAndrews, PJ. Hair transplant goals based on natural patterns of hair loss. In: Hair Transplantation (Series in Cosmetic and Laser Therapy). 5th Edition (Unger WP, Shapiro R, Unger R, Unger M, editors). Thieme Publishers, Stuttgart, 2011; pp. 152–163.

6. McAndrews PJ. Hair transplants in young men. In: Hair Transplant 360. Advances, Techniques, Business Development & Global Perspectives. 1st Edition (Lam S, editor). Jaypee Brothers Medical Publishers, New Delhi, India, 2014; 737–746.

7. Finasteride Male Pattern Hair Loss Study Group. Long-Term 5 Year Multinational Experience with Finasteride 1mg in the Treatment of Men with Androgenetic Alopecia. Eur J Dermatol 2002; 12(1): 38–49.

8. Bernstein RM, Rassman WR. The Aesthetics of Follicular Transplantation. Dermatol Surg 1997; 23(9): 785–799.

22

Miscellaneous Procedures: Intense Pulsed Light, Photodynamic Therapy, Cryotherapy, Cryolipolysis, Microdermabrasion, Salabrasion, Dermabrasion, Microneedling, Radiofrequency, and Ultrasound

Jennifer A. Ledon and Richard G. Bennett

Introduction

Dermatologists are trained to use several devices for removing skin lesion and improving the cosmetic appearance of patients. Whereas some of these devices have been used for many years, others represent new technologies. Often these tools are minimally invasive, efficacious, and have little recovery time.

I. Intense Pulsed Light (IPL)[1,2]

  A. A filtered flashlamp

  B. Emits pulses of divergent light delivered to skin via a sapphire or quartz tip

  C. Noncoherent, broadband light with wavelengths from 515 to 1200 nm. Therefore, cannot be tightly focused like a laser

  D. Effective in treating various skin conditions because it targets all skin chromophores (melanin, water, hemoglobin). This operates under the principle of selective photothermolysis

  E. Compared to lasers which emit coherent monochromatic wavelengths, IPL has variable efficacy and greater side effects

  F. Optical filters in IPL systems can narrow the range of wavelengths transmitted and thus be more selective in targeting melanin, hemoglobin, or water. Shorter wavelengths (515–550 nm) are useful for superficial lesions and patients with light skin; longer wavelengths (700–900 nm) are useful for deep lesions and patients with dark skin. Filters from 500 to 700 nm specifically target melanin. Optical filters can also be used to transmit wavelengths at two different peaks and thus target two types of lesions at one time, e.g., vascular and pigmented lesions

  G. Rectangular and larger spot size (120–450 mm^2) than lasers. This allows efficient treatment of large areas such as the back or chest, but handpiece is bulky and heavy compared to the laser handpiece

  H. Like lasers, both fluence and pulse width are adjustable and help to target certain lesions

  I. Indications for IPL include the following

   1. Fine lines and wrinkles: concomitant use of aminolevulinic acid helps improvement.[3]

   2. Acne scarring.

   3. Hair removal – not as effective as lasers.[4]

    a. Optical filters can minimize epidermal thermal injury from melanin in the epidermis and target melanin in the hair bulb.

4. Vascular lesion removal.

   a. IPL can target oxyhemoglobin, deoxyhemoglobin, and methemoglobin concurrently because of its polychromaticity. Thus, it is very useful for angiomas and rosacea.

5. Pigmented lesion removal.

   a. Useful for melasma and lentigines.[5] Often used in addition to a photoprotective cream and a topical depigmenting agents (e.g., hydroquinone). Usually requires more than one treatment for adequate response.

6. Photorejuvenation.[3]

   a. Improves dyschromia.

7. Poikiloderma of Civatte.

   a. Because it targets melanocytes and blood vessels at the same time, it is effective in eliminating telengiectasias and hyperpigmentation associated with poikiloderma of Civatte.

J. Side effects

1. Dyspigmentation.

   a. Hypopigmentation or hyperpigmentation can occur. These pigmentary changes are due to epidermal injury as IPL emits a broad range of wavelengths and targets more than one chromophore. Pigmentary changes occur in darker skinned or tanned individuals. Stripe type pigmentary alterations can occur but usually fade. To minimize these side effects, patients are advised to avoid sun exposure for 1 week before and after the procedure.

   > Geometrically shaped dyspigmentation after IPL may be very debilitating to patients

2. Pain.

   a. Slight burning or stinging may occur.

3. Erythema.

   a. Mild redness lasting up to 3 days often occurs.

4. Edema.

   a. Usually lasts 1–3 days. If severe, can lead to dyspigmentation or scarring.

5. Purpura.

   a. Unexpected and results from a high energy per unit area (fluence) or a short pulse duration (pulse width).

   b. In contrast to a vascular laser, with IPL purpura does not indicate effective treatment.

II. Photodynamic Therapy (PDT)

A. Requires application of a photosensitizing medication such as aminolevulinic acid (Levulan®) that is activated by a light source (e.g., light-emitting diodes [LED] or IPL)

B. Once activated, the photosensitizer causes a cytotoxic reaction that destroys tissue with the highest photosensitizer concentration. The photosensitizer is particularly concentrated in sebaceous glands and actinically damaged cells

C. Approved by the Food and Drug Administration (FDA) for nonhyperkeratotic actinic keratoses

D. Useful to treat broad areas with multiple actinic keratoses, such as the forehead and scalp, in one sitting

E. May be used off-label combined with nonablative lasers for skin rejuvenation and to decrease wrinkles[6]

F. Must avoid direct sun exposure until treated lesions are healed, usually 1–2 weeks

G. Side effects – pain

III. Cryotherapy[7]

    A. Currently used for the treatment of benign and precancerous skin lesions

> Due to melanocyte sensitivity to cold, care should be taken in patients with dark skin types due to high risk of hypopigmentation.

    B. Liquid nitrogen is the most commonly used medical cryogenic agent, with a boiling point of $-196°C$. It is applied with a cotton-tipped applicator (Figure 3.1A) or with a spray gun (Figure 3.1B)

    C. Lesion destruction is dependent on the freeze-thaw cycle, with cellular damage occurring during the thaw phase. The duration and number of applications needed to successfully destroy a lesion vary and are heavily user dependent

    D. Anesthesia is not required; however, temporary pain and blistering are expected

    E. Average temperatures necessary for destruction are listed below

Target	Temperature Needed for Destruction
Melanocytes	$-5°C$
Benign lesions	$-25°C$
Warts	$-40°C$
Malignant lesions	$-50°C$

IV. Cryolipolysis

    A. Noninvasive body contouring device utilizing cold to selectivity destroy adipocytes

    B. Developed based on the philosophy of "popsicle panniculitis", where prolonged contact with cold popsicles on the buccal mucosa was discovered to lead to panniculitis and, subsequently, fat atrophy

    C. Appropriate patient selection is required

        1. Cryolipolysis is not to be used for overall weight loss or reduction of visceral fat.

        2. Ideal patients are those with small amounts of subcutaneous fat easily gripped by the treatment device handpiece.

    D. Potential side effects

        1. Prolonged neuropathic pain.[8]

        2. Nerve injury.[9]

        3. Paradoxical lipohypertrophy.[10]

        4. Fibrosing disorders, such as morphea.[11]

V. Microdermabrasion[12]

    A. Used for acne, acne scars, stretch marks, photodamage, dyschromia, melasma, and superficial wrinkles

    B. Removes upper layers of epidermis

    C. Uses closed-loop negative pressure system with aluminum oxide or diamond crystals with vacuum removal

    D. Requires eye protection as crystals can cause corneal abrasion

    E. Outcome depends on number of passes on skin and contact time

    F. Usually associated with mild erythema postprocedure

    G. Generally painless with no downtime

VI. Salabrasion

    A. Useful to remove tattoos

    B. Requires table salt and water, each in a separate beaker

    C. Gauze is rolled and held with one hand. The end of the gauze roll is dipped in water and then in salt and then rubbed on the skin in a circular motion until pinpoint bleeding occurs

    D. Aluminum acetate dressing changes are done three times a day followed by antibiotic ointment until wound healing occurs

    E. If done too vigorously may result in scarring

VII. Dermabrasion

    A. Used for acne scarring, postsurgical scarring, fine lines and wrinkles, photoaging, vitiligo, benign lesion removal (e.g., multiple actinic keratoses), and tattoos

    B. Mechanically removes epidermis and superficial dermis. Results in pinpoint bleeding from superficial dermis

    C. Realigns collagen and replaces type III collagen with type I collagen

    D. Done with round wheel with a rough surface. Usually, the wheel with the rough surface is referred to as a diamond fraise (fraise is strawberry in French), which is graded as fine, medium, or course. The fraise is shaped either as a wheel or pear (Figure 22.1). The latter is very effective in reaching into crevasses. The diamond fraise is attached to a motorized handpiece that rotates the wheel

Dermabrasion, although very useful and inexpensive, has been largely replaced by laser treatment.

    E. Alternative types of wheels have a wire brush that penetrates deeper and causes more damage than the diamond fraise

    F. Sandpaper can also be used in lieu of the diamond fraise. The advantage is that this does not require a special motorized instrument. However, sandpaper does not allow easy penetration into crevasses or contours

    G. May be performed on the whole face, a cosmetic unit such as the nose, or on a small area (spot dermabrasion)

       1. Full-face dermabrasion: rarely performed today. Results in edema with a transudate and oozing for 24 hours and erythema for 2–3 weeks or longer. Requires aluminum oxide solution (Burrow's solution) soaks three times a day followed by an antibiotic ointment and nonstick dressing until healing occurs usually in one week. A hydrogel dressing (e.g., Vigilon®) is useful for the first few days because of its cooling effect.

    H. Scarring and permanent hypo- or hyperpigmentation are possible side effects with dermabrasion. Therefore, careful patient selection is necessary. Problems associated with dermabrasion include pain, prolonged erythema, superficial cutaneous infection, milia formation, and reactivation of herpes simplex. Also, differential pigmentation may occur between the dermabraded and nondermabraded skin (pseudohyperpigmentation), which is avoided by feathering the edges

    I. Patients with a history of herpes simplex infection should be given preoperative prophylaxis with acyclovir

    J. Patients who have been on isotretinoin within 12 months should not have dermabrasion[13]

VIII. Microneedling[14,15]

    A. Technique of mechanically creating multiple pinpoint punctures into the skin with needles of various predetermined lengths

Microneedling may be a successful means of transdermal drug delivery in the future.

    B. Uses very fine needles (approximately 0.07 mm in diameter)

    C. Two devices are available

       1. Dermaroller: has very small needles of fixed length distributed along a rolling wand.

       2. Microneedling pen: uses similarly sized needles that oscillate rapidly in and out of the pen that is passed over skin (Figure 22.2). The needle length may be adjusted.

(a)

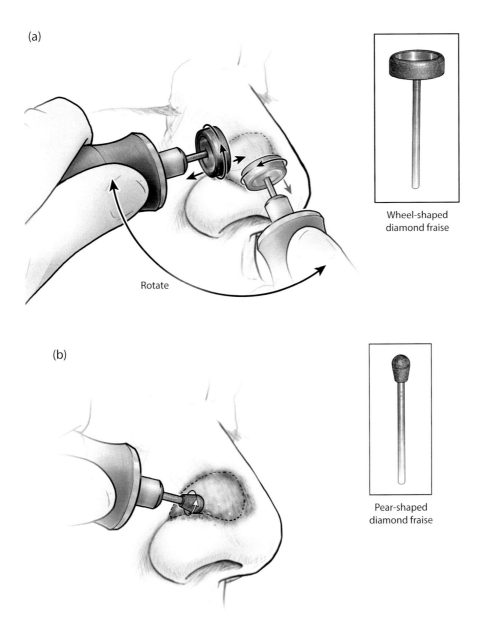

Rotate

Wheel-shaped
diamond fraise

(b)

Pear-shaped
diamond fraise

FIGURE 22.1 Dermabrasion with (A) wheel-shaped diamond fraise and (B) pear-shaped diamond fraise. Note when using the wheel-shaped diamond fraise, one pushes the wheel back and forth perpendicular to the plane of the wheel.

D. Penetration depth ranges from 0.25 to 2.5 mm. Needle length based on anatomic area or skin/scar thickness
  1. Punctures less than 1 mm usually confined to epidermis, do not cause bleeding.
  2. Punctures less than 0.5 mm are painless.
  3. Punctures greater than 1 mm require topical anesthetic and are used for scar improvement and skin rejuvenation.

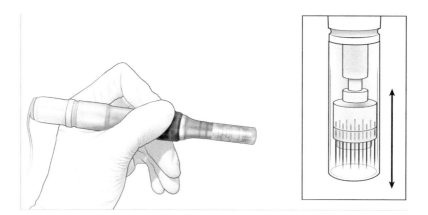

FIGURE 22.2 Microneedling handpiece. Multiple needles move in and out of the skin simultaneously driven by a motor in the handpiece.

    E.   Releases growth factors such as platelet-derived growth factor and fibroblast growth factor that stimulate collagen production

    F.   Indications: acne scarring, striae distensae, scarring, rhytides, melasma, and transdermal drug delivery.[16] Drugs delivered by microneedling include: corticosteroids for alopecia areata, platelet-rich plasma and minoxidil for androgenetic alopecia,[17] photosensitizer + UV light for actinic keratoses and for vitiligo corticosteroids, calcipotriene, topical calcineurin inhibitors, and 5-fluorouracil[18]

    G.   Side effects: pain, bleeding, peeling, foreign body reaction[19]

    H.   Contraindications: active herpes labialis, superficial skin infections

IX. Radiofrequency[20,21]

    A.   Introduces alternating electric current into tissue that creates heat due to the skin resistance to current flow (impedance). This heat is concentrated in the dermis where it results in mild collagen production or skin tightening by collagen contraction. Can be used on all skin types

    B.   Tissue heating is controlled by the electrode type, amount of current, current duration, and cooling time

    C.   Available devices are

        1.   Noninvasive: rests on top of epidermis.

        2.   Noninvasive but fractional: targets tissue in mid to deep dermis.

        3.   Minimally invasive: combined with microneedling or subcutaneous probe (either insulated or noninsulated).

        4.   May be combined with IPL. After IPL is used, tissue is warmer and more sensitive to radiofrequency.

    D.   Indications

        1.   Skin tightening (aka soft tissue coagulation) – improves slightly.

           a.   Neck, jowls, cellulite, abdominal skin.

        2.   Body contouring.

           a.   Decreases excessive fat on abdomen, upper arm, and medial thigh.

        3.   Acne scarring.

        4.   Striae distensae.

        5.   Vaginal rejuvenation.[22,23]

        6.   Axillary osmidrosis and hyperhidrosis.[24]

           a.   Thermal injury to eccrine and apocrine glands reduces sweat and odor.

      7. Endovenous thermal ablation.

         a. Catheter with insulated electrode placed in vein. Radiofrequency energy-generated heat applied to vein wall results in endothelial destruction and subsequent vein occlusion.

   E. Side effects: pain, dysesthesia, erythema, edema, scabbing, thermal burns, fat necrosis. Cutaneous depression from multiple passes or energy too high

X. Ultrasound

   A. High-intensity microfocused sound waves create heat into deep dermis and subcutaneous tissue

   B. Stimulates collagen formation resulting in dermal and subcutaneous tightening

   C. Can disrupt fat cells causing them to dissolve gradually

   D. Can target deeper tissue without affecting superficial tissue; thus spares epidermis from damage

   E. Indications: noninvasive eyebrow elevation, submental and neck tightening, décolletage (low neckline) rejuvenation, body contouring[25],[26]

   F. Side effects

      1. Pain. Anxiolytics and pain medicine often required for treatment.

      2. Erythema.

      3. Edema.

      4. Bruising.

      5. Postinflammatory hypo- or hyperpigmentation.

      6. Numbness or dysesthesia.

      7. Necrosis.

   G. Can be combined with other injectables such as botulinum toxin and fillers. Skin tightening usually performed first

Conclusion

Dermatology and dermatologic surgery continue to be ever-growing fields with not only new technologies, but also the combination and repurposing of existing technologies for a myriad of novel indications. While this chapter serves to introduce a few of these miscellaneous techniques, it is important to keep abreast of new technologies as the fields of dermatology and aesthetics are ever-evolving to help those seeking improvement not only in function and aesthetics, but also in quality of life.

REFERENCES

Intense Pulsed Light (IPL)

1. Babilas P, Schreml S, Szeimies RM, Landthaler M. Intense Pulsed Light (IPL): A Review. Lasers Surg Med 2010; 42: 93–104.
2. Goldberg DJ. Current Trends in Intense Pulsed Light. J Clin Aesthet Dermatol 2012; 5(6): 45–53.
3. Goldman MP, Weiss RA, Weiss MA. Intense Pulsed Light as a Nonablative Approach to Photoaging. Derm Surg 2005; 31(9 (Part 2)): 1179–1187.
4. Fayne RA, Perper M, Eber AE, Aldahan AS, Nouri K. Laser and Light Treatments for Hair Reduction in Fitzpatrick Skin Types IV-VI: A Comprehensive Review of the Literature. Am J Clin Dermatol 2018; 19(2): 237–252.
5. Trivedi MK, Yang FC, Cho BK. A Review of Laser and Light Therapy in Melasma. Int J Womens Dermatol 2017; 3(1): 11–20.

Photodynamic Therapy (PDT)

6. Le Pillouer-Prost A, Cartier H. Photodynamic Photorejuvenation: A Review. Derm Surg 2016; 42(1): 21–30.

Cryotherapy

7. Kuflick EG, Kuflik JH. Cryosurgery. In: Dermatology. 3rd Edition (Bolognia JL, Jorizzo JL, Schaffer JV, editors). Elsevier/Saunders, Philadelphia, PA, 2012; Chapter 138, 2283–2288.

Cryolipolysis

8. Gregory A, Humphrey S, Varas G, Zachary C, Carruthers J. Atypical Pain Developing Subsequent to Cryolipolysis for Noninvasive Reduction of Submental Fat. Derm Surg 2019; 45(3): 487–489.
9. Lee NY, Ibrahim O, Arndt KA, Dover JS. Marginal Mandibular Injury After Treatment With Cryolipolysis. Derm Surg 2018; 44(10): 1353–1355.
10. Stefani WA. Adipose Hypertrophy Following Cryolipolysis. Aesthet Surg J 2015; 35(7): 218–220.
11. Ladha M, Poelman S. Cryolipolysis-Induced Morphea. JAAD Case Rep 2019; 5(4): 300–302.

Dermabrasion

12. Alkhawam L, Alam M. Dermabrasion and Microdermabrasion. Facial Plast Surg 2009; 25(5): 301–310.
13. Waldman A, Bolotin D, Arndt KA, Dover JS, Geronemus RG, Chapas A, Iyengar S et al. ASDS Guidelines Task Force: Consensus Recommendations Regarding the Safety of Lasers, Dermabrasion, Chemical Peels, Energy Devices, and Skin Surgery During and After Isotretinoin Use. Derm Surg 2017; 43 (10): 1249–1262.

Microneedling

14. Alster TS, Graham PM. Microneedling: A Review and Practical Guide. Dermetol Surg 2018; 44(3): 397–404.
15. Bonati LM, Epstein GK, Strugar TL. Microneedling in All Skin Types: A Review. J Drugs Dermatol 2017; 1(16): 308–313.
16. Ibrahim ZA, Hassan GF, Elgendy HY, Al-Shenawy HA. Evaluation of the Efficacy of Transdermal Drug Delivery of Calcipotriol Plus Betamethasone Versus Tacrolimus in the Treatment of Vitiligo. J Cosmetic Dermatol 2019; 18(2): 581–588.
17. Fertig RM, Gamret AC, Cervantes J, Tosti A. Microneedling for the Treatment of Hair Loss? J Eur Acad Dermatol Venereol 2018; 32(4): 564–569.
18. Jha AK, Sonthalia S. 5 Fluorouracil as an Adjuvant Therapy Along with Microneedling in Vitiligo. J Am Acad Dermatol 2019; 80(4): e75–e76.
19. Soltani-Arabshahi R, Wong JW, Duffy KL, Powell DL. Facial Allergic Granulomatous Reaction and Systemic Hypersensitivity Associated with Microneedle Therapy for Skin Rejuvenation. JAMA Dermatol 2014; 150(1): 68–72.

Radiofrequency

20. Levy AS, Grant RT, Rothaus KO. Radiofrequency Physics for Minimally Invasive Aesthetic Surgery. Clin Plast Surg 2016; 43: 551–556.
21. Man J, Goldberg DJ. Safety and Efficacy of Fractional Bipolar Radiofrequency Treatment in Fitzpatrick Skin Types V-VI. J Cosmet Laser Ther 2012; 14(4): 179–183.
22. Hashim PW, Nia JK, Zade J, Farberg AS, Goldenberg G. Noninvasive Vaginal Rejuvenation. Cutis 2018; 102(4): 243–246.
23. Vanaman Wilson MJ, Bolton J, Jones IT, Wu DC, Calame A, Goldman MP. Histologic and Clinical Changes in Vulvovaginal Tissue After Treatment With a Transcutaneous Temperature-Controlled Radiofrequency Device. Dermetol Surg 2018; 44(5): 705–713.
24. Cho SB, Park J, Zheng Z, Yoo KH, Kim H. Split-Axilla Comparison Study of 0.5-MHz, Invasive, Bipolar Radiofrequency Treatment Using Insulated Microneedle Electrodes for Primary Axillary Hyperhidrosis. Skin Res Technol 2019; 25(1): 30–39.

Ultrasound

25. Fabi SG, Burgess C, Carruthers A, Carruthers J, Day D, Goldie K, Pavicic T et al. Consensus Recommendations for Combined Aesthetic Interventions Using Botulinum Toxin, Fillers, and Microfocused Ultrasound in the Neck, Décolletage, Hands, and Other Areas of the Body. Dermetol Surg 2016; 42: 1199–1208.
26. Gutowski KA. Microfocused Ultrasound for Skin Tightening. Clin Plast Surg 2016; 43: 577–582.

Index

Note: Locators in *italics* represent figures and **bold** indicate tables in the text.